T0259284

Sleep Medicine and Dentistry

Guest Editors

RONALD ATTANASIO, DDS, MSEd, MS
DENNIS R. BAILEY, DDS

DENTAL CLINICS OF NORTH AMERICA

www.dental.theclinics.com

April 2012 • Volume 56 • Number 2

SAUNDERS an imprint of ELSEVIER, Inc.

W.B. SAUNDERS COMPANY
A Division of Elsevier Inc.

1600 John F. Kennedy Boulevard • Suite 1800 • Philadelphia, Pennsylvania 19103-2899

http://www.dental.theclinics.com

DENTAL CLINICS OF NORTH AMERICA Volume 56, Number 2
April 2012 ISSN 0011-8532, ISBN 978-1-4557-3849-6

Editor: Yonah Korngold; y.korngold@elsevier.com

Dental Clinics of North America (ISSN 0011-8532) is published quarterly by Elsevier Inc., 360 Park Avenue South, New York, NY 10010-1710. Months of issue are January, April, July, and October. Business and Editorial Offices: 1600 John F. Kennedy Boulevard, Suite 1800, Philadelphia, PA 19103-2899. Periodicals postage paid at New York, NY and additional mailing offices. Subscription prices are $259.00 per year (domestic individuals), $447.00 per year (domestic institutions), $122.00 per year (domestic students/residents), $310.00 per year (Canadian individuals), $563.00 per year (Canadian institutions), $375.00 per year (international individuals), $563.00 per year (international institutions), and $184.00 per year (international and Canadian students/residents). International air speed delivery is included in all *Clinics* subscription prices. All prices are subject to change without notice. **POSTMASTER:** Send address changes to *Dental Clinics of North America*, Elsevier Health Sciences Division, Subscription Customer Service, 3251 Riverport Lane, Maryland Heights, MO 63043. **Customer Service (orders, claims, online, change of address): Elsevier Health Sciences Division, Subscription Customer Service, 3251 Riverport Lane, Maryland Heights, MO 63043. Tel: 1-800-654-2452 (U.S. and Canada). Fax: 314-447-8029. E-mail: journalscustomer service-usa@elsevier.com (for print support); journalsonlinesupport-usa@elsevier.com (for online support)**.

Reprints. For copies of 100 or more, of articles in this publication, please contact the Commercial Reprints Department, Elsevier Inc., 360 Park Avenue South, New York, NY 10010-1710. Tel.: 212-633-3812; Fax: 212-462-1935; E-mail: reprints@elsevier.com.

The *Dental Clinics of North America* is covered in *MEDLINE/PubMed (Index Medicus)*, *Current Contents/Clinical Medicine*, *ISI/BIOMED* and *Clinahl*.

Printed and bound by CPI Group (UK) Ltd, Croydon, CR0 4YY

Transferred to Digital Print 2012

Contributors

GUEST EDITORS

RONALD ATTANASIO, DDS, MSEd, MS
University of Nebraska College of Dentistry, Lincoln, Nebraska

DENNIS R. BAILEY, DDS
Visiting Lecturer, Orofacial Pain and Dental Sleep Medicine; Co-Director, Dental Sleep Medicine Mini-Residency, UCLA School of Dentistry, Los Angeles, California; Private Practice, Denver, Colorado

AUTHORS

FERNANDA ALMEIDA, DDS, PhD
Assistant Professor, Department of Oral Health Sciences, University of British Columbia, Vancouver, British Columbia, Canada

RONALD ATTANASIO, DDS, MSEd, MS
University of Nebraska College of Dentistry, Lincoln, Nebraska

DENNIS R. BAILEY, DDS
Visiting Lecturer, Orofacial Pain and Dental Sleep Medicine; Co-Director, Dental Sleep Medicine Mini-Residency, UCLA School of Dentistry, Los Angeles, California; Private Practice, Denver, Colorado

TERI J. BARKOUKIS, MD
Director, Sleep Medicine Fellowship; Professor of Medicine, Division of Pulmonary, Critical Care, Sleep and Allergy, University of Nebraska Medical Center, Omaha, Nebraska

SABIN R. BISTA, MBBS, FAASM
Associate Director, Sleep Medicine Fellowship; Assistant Professor of Medicine, Division of Pulmonary, Critical Care, Sleep and Allergy, University of Nebraska Medical Center, Omaha, Nebraska

MARIA CLOTILDE CARRA, DMD
PhD Candidate, Faculty of Dental Medicine, Univeristé de Montréal, Montreal, Quebec, Canada

JOHN HARRINGTON, MD, MPH
Associate Professor of Medicine, Division of Sleep Medicine, National Jewish Health, Denver, Colorado

DAVID C. HATCHER, DDS, MSc
Clinical Professor, University of Southern Nevada, Henderson, Nevada; Adjunct Associate Clinical Professor, Arthur A. Dugoni School of Dentistry, San Francisco; Private Practice, Diagnostic Digital Imaging, Sacramento, California

NELLY HUYNH, PhD
Faculty of Dental Medicine, Univeristé de Montréal, Montreal, Quebec, Canada

OFER JACOBOWITZ, MD, PhD
Assistant Professor, New York Presbyterian Hospital, Columbia University; Attending, Mount Sinai Medical Center, New York; Hudson Valley Ear, Nose & Throat PC, Middletown, New York

GILLES LAVIGNE, DMD, PhD, FRDC
Dean of the Faculty of Dental Medicine, Univeristé de Montréal, Montreal, Quebec, Canada

TEOFILO LEE-CHIONG, MD
Professor of Medicine, Chief, Division of Sleep Medicine, National Jewish Health, Denver, Colorado

MARTY R. LIPSEY, DDS, MS
Dental Sleep Med Systems, Inc., Los Angeles; Modesto, California

ROBERT L. MERRILL, DDS, MS
Clinical Professor, UCLA School of Dentistry, Los Angeles, California

BENJAMIN T. PLISKA, DDS, MS, FRCD(C)
Assistant Professor, Department of Oral Health Sciences, University of British Columbia, Vancouver, British Columbia, Canada

T. TROY STENTZ, BA, RPSGT
Clinical Director, Somnos Sleep Disorders Center, Lincoln, Nebraska

JOHN F. TRAPP, MD
Medical Director, Somnos Sleep Disorders Center, Lincoln, Nebraska

Contents

> Sleep medicine as it is known today actually started as research and scientific study, not as clinical medicine. When one considers that sleep medicine today is in its infancy, it is obvious that there is much more to learn. The history of sleep dates back to the 1880s. However, the most significant developments that moved sleep forward into the practice of medicine, and eventually dentistry, occurred from the 1950s on. This article explores the highlights of the history of sleep and sleep medicine.

> Sleep can be defined as a complex reversible state characterized by behavioral quiescence, diminished responsiveness to external stimuli, and a stereotypical species-specific posture. Both components of sleep, non–rapid eye movement and rapid eye movement, are generated and maintained by central nervous system networks that use specific neurotransmitters located in specific areas of the brain. Widespread changes in physiologic processes occur during sleep, and these changes may influence the presentation and severity of specific medical disorders.

> The dentist is well positioned to screen for patients at risk for a sleep disorders, most often a sleep related breathing disorder, and when adequately trained, can treat those diagnosed with sleep apnea using an oral appliance. This treatment requires some degree of training to be able to recognize the symptoms related to the more common sleep disorders. The dentist must determine if the patient is at risk for a sleep disorder through the use of screening questionnaires, reviewing the health history, and additional questioning of the patient.

> Imaging plays a role in the anatomic assessment of the airway and adjacent structures. This article discusses the use of 3-dimensional (3D) imaging (cone beam computed tomography [CBCT]) to evaluate the airway and selected regional anatomic variables that may contribute to obstructive sleep-disordered breathing (OSDB) in patients. CBCT technology uses a cone-shaped x-ray beam with a special image intensifier and a solid-state

sensor or an amorphous silicon plate for capturing the image. Incorporation of 3D imaging into daily practice will allow practitioners to readily evaluate and screen patients for phenotypes associated with OSDB.

John F. Trapp and T. Troy Stentz

The intent of this article is to familiarize dental professionals with the polysomnogram (PSG). The evaluation of patients presenting with sleep disorders is complex, requiring an investigative approach that synthesizes information obtained through a detailed history, a focused physical examination, and appropriate confirmatory testing. The PSG is the only clinical tool that measures multiple physiologic variables to qualitatively and quantitatively evaluate sleep. A proper understanding of the role of the PSG and its measurements and interpretation allows for a proper diagnosis so as to provide an optimal range of treatments for individual patients.

Sabin R. Bista and Teri J. Barkoukis

Normal-sleeping individuals experience a lower metabolic rate and relative cardiovascular quiescent state with lower heart rate and blood pressure that naturally occurs during sleep compared with the waking state. In patients with obstructive sleep apnea (OSA), this quiescent state becomes disrupted. Research has shown a higher risk for several medical disorders, most ominous being a myocardial infarction or stroke. This article serves as an overview to the cardiovascular, cerebrovascular, metabolic, and gastroesophageal effects of OSA.

Maria Clotilde Carra, Nelly Huynh, and Gilles Lavigne

Sleep bruxism (SB) is a common sleep-related motor disorder characterized by tooth grinding and clenching. SB diagnosis is made on history of tooth grinding and confirmed by polysomnographic recording of electromyographic (EMG) episodes in the masseter and temporalis muscles. The typical EMG activity pattern in patients with SB is known as rhythmic masticatory muscle activity (RMMA). The authors observed that most RMMA episodes occur in association with sleep arousal and are preceded by physiologic activation of the central nervous and sympathetic cardiac systems. This article provides a comprehensive review of the cause, pathophysiology, assessment, and management of SB.

Robert L. Merrill

Treatment of sleep apnea with mandibular advancement devices (MADs) may be associated with the development of symptoms of temporomandibular disorder (TMD). This article discusses the different types of TMD and orofacial pain problems that may occur during treatment of obstructive sleep apnea (OSA) with a MAD. It is critical that the general dentist who is providing dental devices for OSA perform a thorough physical and neurologic assessment of the temporomandibular joint and associated structures before providing such a device so that preexisting problems are identified and discussed with the patient.

Oral appliances (OAs) are a primary treatment option for snoring and mild to moderate obstructive sleep apnea (OSA) and are implemented as a noninvasive alternative for patients with severe OSA who are unwilling or unable to tolerate continuous positive airway pressure for the management of their disease. Studies have demonstrated the ability of OAs to eliminate or significantly reduce the symptoms of OSA and produce a measurable influence on the long-term health effects of the disease. Most studies have evaluated one type of OAs, the mandibular advancement splints. This article describes the effectiveness and outcomes of mandibular advancement splints.

The potential use of a portable monitor to assess the outcome of treatment with an oral appliance would ideally be performed by the dentist who is managing the patient's sleep-disordered breathing. Portable monitoring is one of the most cost-effective ways to assess the response to the oral appliance, to determine if further adjustment to the appliance is needed, and to retest to determine the current status following any adjustment. This article emphasizes the use of portable monitors primarily for follow-up care and assessment as opposed to diagnosis or, as it is sometimes referred to, screening.

Positive airway pressure can be effective for OSA treatment but is not effectively used by many patients. Surgical reconstruction of the airway is appropriate for patients who are not otherwise effectively treated or as first-line treatment for patients with focal airway lesions. For surgical planning, examination schemes of the awake patient, as well as sleep endoscopy may be used. Nasal surgery may facilitate treatment using positive airway pressure or oral appliances or to improve quality of life. Pharyngoplasty and tongue base techniques for therapeutic upper airway reconstruction may be performed staged or simultaneously. Current and future approaches are described.

Over the last 5 to 7 years, dental teams have mastered the art and science of processing dental insurance for their patients but have major difficulties learning how to help their patients when it comes to medical insurance. This article attempts to provide a basic guide for the dental team in coding, billing, and processing of major medical insurance for dental sleep medicine. Although there is certainly a learning curve for the dental team in this endeavor, the "patient and physician friendly" dental sleep medicine practice is a model that will help to assure growth and success.

THE CLINICS ARE NOW AVAILABLE ONLINE!

Access your subscription at:
www.theclinics.com

Preface

Sleep Medicine in Dentistry

This issue of the *Dental Clinics of North America* is designed to enlighten the reader about the current status of various topics in sleep medicine that are of interest to the dentist. The overall intent is for this text to explore various aspects of sleep medicine that are or may be common in the everyday practice of dentistry.

SECTION I: INTRODUCTION TO SLEEP MEDICINE

This is a basic overview and introduction to sleep and sleep medicine. The focus is on sleep-related breathing disorders (snoring and sleep apnea) because this is the most common sleep disorder that involves the dentist, from the standpoint of recognition as well as treatment. The dentist who becomes involved in the treatment of sleep apnea patients will need to become aware of other sleep disorders as well. These include insomnia, restless leg syndrome, and periodic limb movement disorders, to name a few. All of these disorders may involve both adults and children; however, it is only recently that attention has been paid to the younger age group. The most common finding is snoring and this may be a sign that the patient is at risk for sleep apnea.

SECTION II: EVALUATION AND RISK ASSESSMENT FOR SLEEP DISORDERS

In this section the assessment of a patient is covered from the standpoint of screening as well as from a more comprehensive aspect. This includes a clinical evaluation of the head, neck, and airway to what the most up-to-date imaging demonstrates to the results of a sleep study and how the dentist would evaluate the findings from such a study.

SECTION III: HEALTH AND MEDICAL CONSEQUENCES OF SLEEP DISORDERS

Sleep apnea and to some degree even snoring has an impact on the health and well-being of the patient. Dentists are involved more than ever in the overall health of the patient. This involves not only the health of the patient but also areas of everyday concern that the dentist sees and may treat. Therefore the need to understand the relationship between common conditions seen by the dentist is important. This includes orofacial pain/temporomandibular disorders as well as bruxism. Sleep disorders and especially sleep breathing disorders have a bidirectional relationship to a wide variety of health-related consequences.

SECTION IV: ORAL APPLIANCES: THERAPY FOR SLEEP-RELATED BREATHING DISORDERS

Oral appliance therapy is becoming more and more accepted for the management of sleep apnea and snoring. Today many patients prefer an alternative to continuous positive airway pressure (CPAP) and most often this is the oral appliance. In 2006

Dent Clin N Am 56 (2012) xi–xiii
doi:10.1016/j.cden.2012.03.002
dental.theclinics.com

the American Academy of Sleep Medicine published the practice parameters for the use of oral appliances and it was determined that the oral appliance is an option for patients who desire it when diagnosed with mild to moderate sleep apnea.[1] In this section, there will be a focus on the current status of oral appliances and their effectiveness. In addition a review of the use of home sleep testing (portable monitors) for the determination of oral appliance effectiveness is reviewed. Last, reimbursement is an issue and this is also reviewed.

SECTION V: OTHER THERAPIES FOR SLEEP-RELATED BREATHING DISORDERS

There are many other ways in which sleep disorders and particularly snoring and sleep apnea may be addressed. CPAP or positive airway pressure has historically been the gold standard for the management of sleep apnea. This text will not cover this since this is a form of therapy most often provided by the sleep medicine physician and is not something the dentist will provide for patients. However it is necessary for the dentist to know about the patient who is using CPAP. The use of CPAP would indicate that a diagnosis of sleep apnea has been made. Sleep apnea is a medical condition and should be acknowledged in a health history. In addition it has been shown that CPAP can have a negative impact on the skeletal structures as well as impact tooth position and even alter the occlusion.[2] Surgery has a role in the management of sleep apnea as well. A wide variety of surgical procedures is available and must be considered based on the anatomic situation being addressed. Many times surgery can also be done adjunctively with CPAP or with an oral appliance. Last, consideration needs to be given to other alternative therapies that can help in the management of snoring and sleep apnea. These include weight loss, better sleeping habits (sleep hygiene), and more exercise. An improved awareness of the importance of sleep can lead to improved quality of life overall. Sleep, not only the quality but also the amount, is just as important as exercise and diet according to the National Sleep Foundation.

CONCLUSION

This text is designed to be informative and to open up a greater awareness of issues encountered by the practicing dentist as it relates to sleep and sleep medicine. There are many textbooks that cover sleep/sleep medicine in a more comprehensive and scientific manner as well as organizations with an interest in sleep medicine and these are reviewed in the Appendix. It is the hope and intent that this text will be enlightening and timely as it relates to a discipline in medicine that has major implications for the involvement of the practicing dentist.

Ronald Attanasio, DDS, MSEd, MS
University of Nebraska College of Dentistry
Lincoln, NE 68583, USA

Dennis R. Bailey, DDS
UCLA School of Dentistry
10833 Le Conte Avenue, CHS-Box 951668
Los Angeles, CA 90095, USA

E-mail addresses:
rattanas@unmc.edu (R. Attanasio)
RMC4E@aol.com (D.R. Bailey)

REFERENCES

1. Kushida CA, Morgenthaler TI, Littner MR, et al. Practice parameters for the treatment of snoring and obstructive sleep apnea with oral appliances: an update for 2005. Sleep 2006;29(2):240–3.
2. Tsuda H, Almeida FR, Tsuda T, et al. Craniofacial changes after 2 years of nasal continuous positive airway pressure use in patients with obstructive sleep apnea. Chest 2010;138(4):870–4.

The History of Sleep Medicine

Dennis R. Bailey, DDS[a,b,*], Ronald Attanasio, DDS, MSEd, MSc[c]

KEYWORDS

• History • Oral appliances • Sleep medicine
• Dental sleep medicine

Sleep medicine as it is known today actually started as research and scientific study, not as clinical medicine. When one considers that sleep medicine today is in its infancy, it is obvious that there is much more to learn. The history of sleep dates back to the 1880s. However, the most significant developments that moved sleep forward into the practice of medicine, and eventually dentistry, occurred from the 1950s on. This article explores the highlights of the history of sleep and sleep medicine.

SLEEP: THE EARLY DAYS

1880 Gelineau, a French neurologist, recognizes narcolepsy and cataplexy as a condition associated with sudden sleep attacks, distinct from epilepsy.[1] This aspect of sleep was the earliest recognized.

1937 Loomis and colleagues[2] document the characteristics on an electroencephalogram of what is now known as NREM (non–rapid eye movement) sleep. Loomis outlines 5 stages of the increasing depth of sleep, classified as A through E.

1953 A new sleep stage called REM (rapid eye movement) sleep is discovered by Dement and Kleitman. This stage of sleep is believed to be associated with dreaming.[3]

1957 Dement and Kleitman[3] propose a new classification of sleep, which proposes 4 stages of NREM sleep as well as REM sleep. These investigators describe how NREM sleep has increasing levels of depth, followed by REM. These 2 stages occur in repeating cycles throughout the night. This description of the sleep cycle continues to be used today, with few changes.

1964 A Narcolepsy Center is established at Stanford University.[4]

1966 Researchers in Europe describe the clinical entity of sleep apnea syndrome. This condition is associated with obstructive apneas and symptoms of daytime

[a] Orofacial Pain and Dental Sleep Medicine, Dental Sleep Medicine Mini-Residency, UCLA School of Dentistry, 10833 Le Conte Avenue, CHS-Box 951668, Los Angeles, CA 90095, USA
[b] Private Practice, Denver, CO, USA
[c] University of Nebraska College of Dentistry, Lincoln, NE 68583, USA
* Corresponding author. 8400 East Prentice Avenue, Suite 804, Greenwood Village, CO 80111.
E-mail address: RMC4E@aol.com

Dent Clin N Am 56 (2012) 313–317
doi:10.1016/j.cden.2012.02.004
0011-8532/12/$ – see front matter © 2012 Elsevier Inc. All rights reserved.

dental.theclinics.com

sleepiness that are often severe. At this point the only treatment is a tracheotomy.[5]

1968 A manual is developed for the scoring of sleep.

THE BEGINNING OF SLEEP AS A MEDICAL DISCIPLINE

In the 1970s sleep medicine started to become integrated in the practice of medicine. Throughout the 1970s there was significant activity that fostered sleep as a medical discipline and not just as a scientific or research field. During this time there was an increased interest by many of the related medical specialties, and sleep medicine as a subspecialty was beginning to take shape.

1970 Stanford University develop the first comprehensive sleep center, and the ability to perform nocturnal polysomnography (sleep study) is developed.

1975 At this time there are now 5 sleep centers. Up until this time sleep medicine has been viewed as experimental. At the same time the need for an organization that would be oriented around the sleep center and that would also provide a medical and research direction is created. The Association of Sleep Disorders Centers (ASDC) is duly founded. This organization today is known as the American Academy of Sleep Medicine (AASM).[4]

1976 The ASDC form a nosology committee to develop a diagnostic system that will consider all of the various sleep and arousal disorders that are seen clinically.

1977 The ASDC accredits the first sleep center at Montefiore Hospital in New York City.

1978 The first issue of the journal *Sleep* is published.

As the organization dedicated to sleep medicine moved into the 1980s and the 1990s, the interest in this field was also growing. Through the 1980s the recognition and prevalence of sleep apnea as well as the treatment formed the basis for the developments over the decades to come. The number of people with an interest in sleep medicine and research was growing at an unprecedented rate. The number of events that occurred over these 2 decades was very significant. In the early 1990s dentistry became involved with sleep and sleep medicine through the establishment of the Sleep Disorders Dental Society.

1980 The first report on the successful use of an oral appliance is published: the tongue-retaining device.[6]

1981 Sullivan and colleagues[7] introduce a new treatment for sleep apnea: continuous positive airway pressure (CPAP). CPAP became the mainstay of treatment in the early days, and has continued to be the gold standard for the management of sleep apnea.

1986 The first scientific meeting dedicated to sleep and sleep disorders is held in Columbus, Ohio. The meeting is attended by more than 700 people and will eventually become an annual event. The meeting is jointly held by the ASDC, the Sleep Research Society (SRS), and the Association of Polysomnographic Technologists (APT), which become known collectively as the Associated Professional Sleep Societies (APSS).[4]

1987 Ancoli-Israel and colleagues use home testing devices, finding that in the 358 people tested, 31% of the men and 19% of the women have sleep apnea.[8]

1987 The ASDC changes its name to the American Sleep Disorders Association (ASDA) and will eventually be known as the AASM.

1988 The first major textbook on sleep entitled *Principles and Practice of Sleep Medicine* is published by Kryger, Roth and Dement.[9]

1989 The AASM begins to accredit fellowship programs in sleep medicine for physicians with an interest in this field.

1990 The first comprehensive publication designed for the diagnosis of sleep disorders is published. It is entitled the *International Classification of Sleep Disorders* (ICSD-1).[10]

1991 Dentistry becomes involved with sleep medicine through the establishment of the Sleep Disorders Dental Society (SDDS). The SDDS is founded by 8 founding members and 26 charter members.

1992 The SDDS develops its bylaws, and is incorporated and has its inaugural meeting in Phoenix, Arizona.

1992 The first practice parameters document is published by the AASM. These articles will continue to be published on a wide variety of topics in sleep medicine as a guideline for the diagnosis and treatment of sleep disorders.

1993 A study is published by Young and colleagues[11] that to this day is cited in numerous publications, which defines the prevalence of sleep apnea in the general population.

1993 The National Center for Sleep Disorders Research and Education is established by the National Institutes of Health.

1994 The American Medical Association (AMA) recognizes sleep medicine as a subspecialty.[12]

1995 The first Practice Parameters for the use of oral appliances is published in the journal *Sleep*.[13]

1996 The American Dental Association (ADA) approves the SDDS educational programs for continuing education.

1998 The first Certification Examination for dentists with advanced training and knowledge in sleep medicine is given.

1999 The ASDA changes its name to the AASM and continues to be known as such up to the present time.

As sleep medicine entered the 2000s, the interest by both physicians and dentists continued to grow. In addition, the recognition of the role of the dentist continued to grow and mature, and this was particularly well recognized in the use of the oral appliance for the management of sleep apnea. Acceptance of oral appliances was beginning to grow after the publication of the practice parameters paper. The number of oral appliances grew through the 1980s and 1990s but seemed to become better recognized in the last decade. At the same time, the interest on the part of the dental professional was also expanding.

2000 A special interest section on oral appliances is established in the AASM. This section has since been incorporated into the section on sleep breathing disorders.

2000 The SDDS becomes the Academy of Dental Sleep Medicine (ADSM).

2003 The ADSM 12th annual meeting is now held in conjunction with the APSS annual sleep meeting.

2004 The American Board of Dental Sleep Medicine (ABDSM) is established. This body replaces the Certification Program that was created in 1998. The ABDSM is a testing and examination group that grants Diplomate status to those who meet the requirements and successfully pass the examination; this is designated as D.ABDSM. As of 2010, there were 161 dentists who had achieved this level.

2006 The ADSM changes its name to the American Academy of Dental Sleep Medicine (AADSM).

2006 The practice parameters for the use of oral appliances are published by the AASM, updating the original publication that appeared in 1995. This updated review significantly improves the validity of oral appliances for the management of sleep apnea and snoring.[14]

2010 The number of AASM-accredited sleep centers for sleep breathing disorders (sleep apnea and snoring) exceeds 2000.

2010 The membership of the AASM exceeds 9000 and the AADSM membership is more than 2200, with 161 D.ABDSMs.

THE FUTURE: 2011 AND BEYOND

Sleep medicine, for the dentist in particular, continues to grow at a rapid pace. More articles appear in journals read by the dentist, and there are more courses at dental meetings and conventions that deal with the dentist's role in sleep disorders, snoring, sleep apnea, sleep bruxism, and oral appliance therapy. The future is bright for the dentist to have an increasingly important role in this field. There will be continued involvement of dentists with their medical colleagues in relation to patient care and the management of sleep apnea and snoring. Regardless, it is important for anyone entering this field to be well trained in a comprehensive way, based on sound evidence.

REFERENCES

1. Schmidt-Nowara W. A review of sleep disorders: the history and diagnosis of sleep disorders related to the dentist. Dent Clin North Am 2001;45(4):632.
2. Loomis AL, Harvey EN, Hobart GA. Cerebral states during sleep as studied by human brain potentials. J Exp Psychol 1937;21:127–44.
3. Dement WC, Kleitman N. Cyclic variations in EEG during sleep and their relation to eye movements, body motility and dreaming. Electroencephalogr Clin Neurophysiol 1957;9:673–90.
4. Shepard JW, Buysee DJ, Chesson AL, et al. History of the development of sleep medicine in the United States. J Clin Sleep Med 2005;1(1):61–82.
5. Gastaut H, Tassinari CA, Duron B, et al. Polygraphic study of the episodic diurnal and nocturnal (hypnic and respiratory) manifestations of the Pickwick syndrome. Brain Res 1966;1(2):167–86.
6. Cartwright RD, Samelson CF. The effects of a nonsurgical treatment for obstructive sleep apnea. JAMA 1982;248:705–9.
7. Sullivan CE, Issa FG, Berthon-Jones M, et al. Reversal of obstructive sleep apnoea by continuous positive airway pressure applied through the nares. Lancet 1981;1(8225):862–5.
8. Ancoli-Israel S, Kripke DF, Mason W. Characteristics of obstructive and central sleep apnea in the elderly: an interim report. Biol Psychiatry 1987;22(6):741–50.
9. Kryger MR, Roth T, Dement WC, editors. Principles and practice of sleep medicine. 4th edition. St Louis (MO): Elsevier Saunders; 2005.
10. International Classification of Sleep Disorders–Second Edition (ICSD-2). Darien (IL): American Academy of Sleep Medicine; 2005.
11. Young T, Palta M, Dempsey J, et al. The occurrence of sleep-related breathing among middle-aged adults. N Engl J Med 1993;328:1230–5.

12. Young T. Rationale, design, and findings from the Wisconsin Sleep Cohort Study: toward understanding the total societal burden of sleep-disordered breathing. Sleep Med Clin 2009;4(1):38.
13. Practice parameters for the treatment of snoring and obstructive sleep apnea with oral appliances. American Sleep Disorders Association. Sleep 1995;18(6):511–3.
14. Kushida CA, Morgenthaler TI, Littner MR, et al; American Academy of Sleep. Practice parameters for the treatment of snoring and obstructive sleep apnea with oral appliances: an update for 2005. Sleep 2006;29(2):240–3.

In addition dates of significant events were found in newsletter publications from the American Academy of Sleep Medicine (AASM) and from the American Academy of Dental Sleep Medicine (AADSM).

Basic Biology of Sleep

John Harrington, MD, MPH*, Teofilo Lee-Chiong, MD

KEYWORDS

• Sleep • REM • NREM • Circadian rhythms

Sleep can be defined as a complex reversible state characterized by behavioral quiescence, diminished responsiveness to external stimuli, and a stereotypical species-specific posture. Unlike other states of reduced awareness and receptivity to environmental influences, such as coma, delirium, or encephalopathy, both components of sleep, non–rapid eye movement (NREM) and rapid eye movement (REM), are generated and maintained by central nervous system (CNS) networks that use specific neurotransmitters located in specific areas of the brain.

CONTROL OF SLEEP AND WAKING

Three physiologic processes control sleep latency (ie, time taken to fall asleep), duration and quality, and alertness, namely, (1) sleep homeostasis, (2) circadian rhythm, and (3) sleep inertia.[1,2] In addition, the timing of sleep and waking is also determined by behavioral influences, such as social activities, meals, and work responsibilities.

Sleep homeostasis is the increase in sleep pressure related to the duration of immediate prior wakefulness. This sleep pressure declines with sustained sleep. Slow wave (delta) activity (SWA) is often used as a marker of homeostatic sleep pressure among adults. Like sleep homeostasis, SWA increases during sustained wakefulness and diminishes after sustained NREM sleep. Thus, it is more difficult to arouse a person when SWA is high. The neurotransmitter adenosine is believed to regulate this homeostatic sleep drive.

The circadian rhythm, on the other hand, is independent of the sleep-wake cycle. Its main function is promoting wakefulness. Most individuals have 2 circadian rhythm–related peaks in alertness, during the late morning and early evening, and 2 periods of circadian troughs in alertness, in the early morning and early midafternoon. Increase in circadian alertness resists the increase in homeostatic sleep pressure during the waking period, and a decreasing circadian alertness opposes the decreasing homeostatic sleep throughout the sleep period, thereby maintaining constant alertness during the biological day and consolidated sleep during the biological night.

Sleep inertia, or a period of relative confusion and disorientation during the transition between sleep and waking, is responsible for the sensation of sleepiness at the start of the biological day when sleep homeostasis is at its lowest level.[2]

Division of Sleep Medicine, National Jewish Health, 1400 Jackson Street, Denver, CO 80206, USA
* Corresponding author.
E-mail address: harringtonj@njhealth.org

Dent Clin N Am 56 (2012) 319–330
doi:10.1016/j.cden.2012.01.005
0011-8532/12/$ – see front matter © 2012 Elsevier Inc. All rights reserved.

dental.theclinics.com

NEUROANATOMY OF SLEEP AND WAKING

The states of wake, NREM sleep, and REM sleep are each generated by discrete but interconnected neural networks that use specific neurotransmitters. There are several key sleep-wake neurotransmitters, including glutamate (main CNS excitatory neurotransmitter), γ-aminobutyric acid (GABA, main NREM neurotransmitter), acetylcholine (main REM sleep neurotransmitter), and glycine (responsible for inhibition of spinal motor neurons that cause muscle atonia during REM sleep).[3]

Main neurotransmitters (and their neurons) involved in generating waking include acetylcholine (basal forebrain and pedunculopontine tegmentum/laterodorsal tegmentum in the brainstem), dopamine (substantia nigra), glutamate (reticular formation, thalamus, and hypothalamus), histamine (tuberomammillary nucleus), hypocretin (lateral hypothalamic perifornical region), norepinephrine (locus coeruleus), and serotonin (dorsal raphe). Main neurotransmitters (and their neurons) involved in the generation of sleep include acetylcholine (for REM sleep), adenosine (basal forebrain), GABA (ventrolateral preoptic region), and melatonin (pineal gland).[4]

Acetylcholine is both a wake and a REM sleep neurotransmitter and is responsible for cortical electroencephalographic (EEG) desynchronization seen during these 2 stages. Cholinergic agonists (eg, physostigmine) increase REM sleep, whereas cholinergic antagonists (eg, tricyclic antidepressants) decrease REM sleep.

Adenosine, a sleep neurotransmitter, is, as stated earlier, responsible for the homeostatically driven sleep pressure. A byproduct of the breakdown of adenosine triphosphate (ATP) released by glutamate-stimulated astrocytes, levels of adenosine progressively increase during prolonged wakefulness and decrease during sleep. Adenosine acts by inhibiting wake-promoting regions of the brain (via A_1 receptors) and activating ventrolateral preoptic nucleus (VLPO) neurons (via A_{2A} receptors). Adenosine receptor blockers (eg, caffeine) increase wakefulness and decrease EEG SWA during sleep.

Dopamine is a wake neurotransmitter; D_1 receptor agonists (eg, amphetamines) that enhance dopamine release increase wakefulness, and dopamine antagonists (haloperidol and chlorpromazine) promote sleep. Glutamate is another wake and REM neurotransmitter, levels of which increase during waking and REM sleep and decrease during NREM sleep. Glutamate stimulates the release of ATP by astrocytes. Histamine, a wake neurotransmitter, is blocked by first-generation histamine-1 receptor blockers (eg, diphenhydramine) and by low-dose doxepin, leading to sedation. GABA agonists (eg, barbiturates, benzodiazepines receptor agonists, and sodium oxybate) cause sedation and sleepiness.

Hypocretin (orexin) promotes wakefulness and suppresses REM sleep, and dysfunction of this neurotransmitter is associated with narcolepsy-cataplexy. Agonists of norepinephrine (eg, isoproterenol), a wake neurotransmitter, increase arousal and wakefulness. Precursors and reuptake inhibitors of serotonin, a wake neurotransmitter, promote wakefulness.

Through their effects on one or more of these neurotransmitters, drugs and substances can be sedating, alerting, or both, because of direct action on the neuronal receptors, adverse reaction, or withdrawal effect. For example, stimulants can prolong sleep onset latency and decrease total sleep time by increasing levels of dopamine and norepinephrine (seen with amphetamine, cocaine, and methylphenidate), by augmenting the actions of hypocretin and dopamine (believed to account for the effects of modafinil and armodafinil), by decreasing adenosine levels (caffeine), or by enhancing acetylcholine release (nicotine). Stimulants, as a class, decrease sleepiness and fatigue, increase alertness, and enhance daytime performance and memory.[5] On the other hand, sedating medications (eg, benzodiazepine receptor agonists express-ing affinity for $GABA_A$ receptors and ramelteon, a melatonin receptor agonist) gener-ally shorten sleep onset latency; long acting formulations of sedating agents may also increase both total sleep time and sleep efficiency (ratio of total sleep time to total time in bed).[6]

Aminergic neurons, activity of which decreases during NREM and REM sleep rela-tive to waking, and cholinergic neurons, which are active during wake and REM sleep, interact to switch between wakefulness and sleep (NREM and REM).

CIRCADIAN RHYTHMS

Biological rhythms are ubiquitous, being present in prokaryotic and eukaryotic microbes, plants, insects, and animals, including humans. These rhythms are charac-terized by specific amplitude (maximal excursion from peak to nadir), peak, nadir, phase, and frequency (number of oscillations per unit time). The term circadian refers to 1 oscillation approximately every 24 hours. Phase is the temporal position of the endogenous rhythm in relation to an external reference, such as the 24-hour light-dark cycle. A phase is considered advanced if it is shifted to an earlier time in the 24-hour cycle or delayed if it occurs later during the cycle. Most intrinsic human circa-dian rhythms are not exactly 24 hours (commonly about 24.2 hours) and tend to free run at this longer frequency in the absence of environmental time cues. The process by which external cues adjust the phase (forward or backward) of the intrinsic circadian rhythms is called entrainment, and the environmental cues that are capable of entrain-ing intrinsic circadian rhythms are referred to as zeitgebers.[7] Light is the dominant zeit-geber, but other factors such as exogenous melatonin and timing of activities are capable of phase shifting intrinsic circadian rhythms. Light provided at night before minimum core body temperature (CTmin) can cause phase delay of the sleep-wake rhythm, and morning light provided after CTmin can cause a phase advance.

The suprachiasmatic nucleus (SCN) is the master circadian rhythm generator in mammals, promoting wakefulness during the day and consolidating sleep during the night. The main afferent pathway involves photic stimuli reaching the retina and from the retina to the SCN via the retinohypothalamic tract.[8] Retinal ganglion cells contain melanopsin and are most sensitive to shorter wavelength light (blue to blue-green). Other photic (GABAergic, histaminergic, and cholinergic) and nonphotic (sero-tonergic) pathways also exist. The SCN has efferent projections to several CNS areas, including the hypothalamus and pineal gland, where melatonin is synthesized and released. Like light exposure, melatonin can influence the sleep-wake rhythm, phase delaying and advancing the rhythm when given in the morning and evening, respectively.

PHYSIOLOGY DURING SLEEP

There are significant changes to several physiologic variables that occur during sleep, including autonomic, respiratory, cardiac, renal/genitourinary, gastrointestinal, endo-crine, thermoregulatory, and immunologic measures.

Autonomic Nervous System

Compared with levels during wake, sympathetic activity diminishes and parasympa-thetic activity increases during NREM sleep; these changes are magnified further during tonic REM sleep. Sympathetic activity transiently increases during phasic REM sleep.[9]

Respiratory System

Although metabolic factors (ie, pH, Pa_{O_2}, and Pa_{CO_2}) and behavioral factors control respiration during wakefulness, the latter is lost during sleep, leaving only metabolic factors to remain operational during sleep. Thus, during early N1 sleep, periodic breathing with episodes of central apneas/hypopneas and hyperpneas can develop as Pa_{CO_2} levels fluctuate below and above the apneic threshold, respectively. Respiration becomes regular in frequency and amplitude during stable N3 sleep but may become irregular again during REM sleep with variable tidal volumes and respiratory rates.[10] Hypoxic and hypercapnic ventilatory responses, upper airway dilator muscle tone, and activity of accessory muscles of respiration decrease during NREM sleep compared with wakefulness and diminish further during REM sleep. Compared with waking levels, Pa_{O_2} levels generally decrease by about 2 to 12 mm Hg, oxygen saturation levels decrease by about 2%, and Pa_{CO_2} levels increase by 2 to 8 mm Hg.

Cardiovascular System

Heart rate, cardiac output, blood pressure (BP), and systemic vascular resistance change with sleep, being relatively lower during NREM and tonic REM sleep than during wakefulness and higher during phasic REM sleep and awakenings than during NREM and tonic REM sleep.[9] In addition, nighttime systolic BP is commonly about 10% less than daytime levels, a phenomenon referred to as BP dipping.[11]

Renal/Genitourinary System

Urine production diminishes during sleep because of reduced glomerular filtration as well as increased water reabsorption and renin release. During REM sleep, penile tumescence may develop in men and clitoral tumescence and vaginal engorgement in women.

Gastrointestinal System

Basal gastric acid secretion displays a circadian rhythmicity, with peak levels between 10 PM and 2 AM and lowest levels between 5 AM and 11 AM. Other sleep-related changes in the gastrointestinal system include decrease in salivary production, swallowing rate, and esophageal and intestinal motility.

Endocrine System

Secretion of hormones is influenced by circadian rhythms, sleep, or both.[12] For instance, cortisol secretion is linked primarily to circadian rhythms, whereas growth hormone (GH) secretion is linked primarily to sleep, specifically N3 sleep. Secretion of thyrotropin, by comparison, is linked to both sleep and circadian rhythms. Levels of GH increase, and levels of both cortisol and adrenocorticotropic hormone (ACTH) decrease during the first half of the sleep period. During the second half of the sleep period, GH levels decrease, whereas cortisol and ACTH levels increase. Release of GH and prolactin occurs primarily during N3 sleep; in contrast, thyrotropin and cortisol secretion is inhibited by sleep.

Thermoregulatory System

Core body temperature generally peaks in the late afternoon and early evening (6 PM–8 PM) and decreases at the onset of sleep, with temperature nadir (4 AM–5 AM) occurring about 2 hours before usual wake time (CTmin). Sleep, itself, is associated with several changes in thermoregulation, namely, decline in core body temperature, decrease in thermal set point, increase in heat loss because of peripheral vasodilatation, and decrease in metabolic heat production with loss of heat generation due to shivering in REM sleep. All these changes result in reduced thermoregulatory responses to thermal challenges. Both sleep quality and architecture are determined by changes in body temperature at bedtime: (1) sleep is suppressed if the individual is exposed to extremely hot or cold environmental temperatures, (2) sleep is enhanced if it is attempted during the falling phase of the temperature rhythm after maximum core body temperature, and (3) waking occurs during the rising phase of the temperature rhythm after CTmin.[13]

Immunologic System

Proinflammatory cytokines, such as interleukin (IL) 1β and tumor necrosis factor α (TNF-α), enhance NREM sleep, whereas anti-inflammatory cytokines, such as IL-4, IL-10, and transforming growth factor β, suppress sleep.[14] Acute infectious and inflammatory processes can give rise to sleepiness due, at least in part, to these changes in immune processes. Obstructive sleep apnea can also be considered an inflammatory disorder because it is associated with increased levels of proinflammatory markers, such as C-reactive protein, IL-6, and TNF-α, as well as decreased levels of anti-inflammatory markers.

MEASUREMENT OF SLEEP

Polysomnography (PSG) is commonly used to objectively characterize sleep and its various stages. PSG consists of continuous and simultaneous recordings of several physiologic variables during the sleep period, such as EEG, electro-oculography (EOG), and chin electromyography (EMG). Other monitors may be used during PSG, including electrocardiography, airflow and snoring sensors, thoracic and abdominal movement detectors, oximetry, and limb EMG, to identify abnormal sleep-related respiratory events, limb movements, or behaviors.[15]

EEG consists of placement of scalp electrodes based on the International 10–20 system, in which each electrode is provided with a letter (region of the brain) and a numerical subscript, such as F (frontal), C (central), O (occipital), M (mastoid), odd numbers (left-sided electrodes), even numbers (right-sided electrodes), and Z (midline electrodes). Using the recommended EEG electrode placements, F4M1, C4M1, and O2M1, the summed potential activity of cortical neurons are recorded as waves of different frequencies (cycles per second or Hz), namely, beta (>13 Hz), alpha (8–13 Hz), theta (4–7 Hz), or delta (<4 Hz). Beta waves are seen during alert wakefulness; alpha waves during waking with eyes closed; theta waves during N1, N2, and REM sleep; and delta waves during N3 sleep.

EOG records the difference in potentials (dipole) between a positively charged cornea and a negatively charged retina. Recommended EOG electrode placements are E1M2 and E2M2, with E referring to the outer canthus of the eye. These electrode locations create voltage changes with eye movements (ie, positive voltage causing a downward tracing deflection when the eye moves toward an electrode and a negative voltage with an upward tracing deflection when the eye moves away from an electrode). Two general patterns of eye movements can often be seen: (1) slow rolling eye movements that are present during waking with closed eyes, N1 sleep, or brief awakenings and (2) REMs that occur during wakefulness with open eyes (eye blinks) or REM sleep.

Chin EMG uses 3 electrodes, one on the midline above the inferior edge of the mandible and one each on either side of the midline below the inferior edge of the mandible.

Sleep is conventionally classified as either NREM or REM sleep. NREM sleep is further subdivided into N1, N2, and N3 sleep. In scoring wake and sleep stages, PSG data are divided into 30-second periods or epochs, and each epoch is assigned a single sleep stage that comprises the greatest percentage of that epoch. An epoch is classified as stage wake if more than 50% of the epoch has alpha EEG waves with eye closure. Other characteristic features include conjugate vertical eye blinks, reading eye movements, voluntary rapid open eye movements, and a relatively high chin EMG tone (**Fig. 1**). When alpha EEG waves are replaced by low-voltage, mixed frequency (4–7 Hz) waves that occupy more than 50% of the epoch, the epoch is scored as stage N1 sleep. In persons in whom alpha waves are not generated, the epoch is considered N1 if the EEG consists of 4- to 7-Hz waves with slowing of activity by 1 Hz or more compared with stage wake. During stage N1 sleep, vertex sharp waves and slow eye movements (but not REMs) may be observed. There are no K complexes and sleep spindles in the EEG tracings, and chin EMG tone is commonly lower than during relaxed wakefulness (**Fig. 2**).

Stage N2 sleep is defined by the presence of either K complexes (high-amplitude biphasic wave with duration of 0.5 seconds or more) or sleep spindles (oscillations with a frequency of 12–14 Hz lasting 0.5–1.5 seconds) during the first half of the epoch or during the last half of the previous epoch, and if criteria for stage N3 (see later) are absent (**Fig. 3**). The epoch is classified as stage N3 sleep if 20% or more of it is occupied by slow wave (0.5–2 Hz and >75 μV) EEG activity (**Fig. 4**). Stage REM consists of low-amplitude mixed-frequency EEG activity, rapid EOG movements, and relatively lower chin EMG tone compared with other sleep stages (**Fig. 5**). Stages N1, N2, N3, and REM typically account for 5%, 45%, 25%, and 25% of total sleep time, respectively, among healthy unmedicated adults.

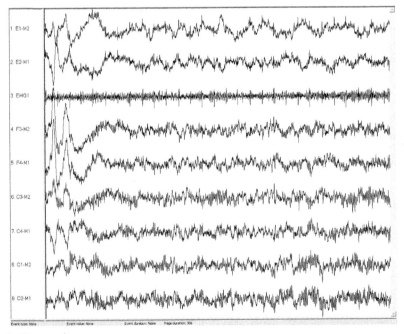

Fig. 1. Stage wake.

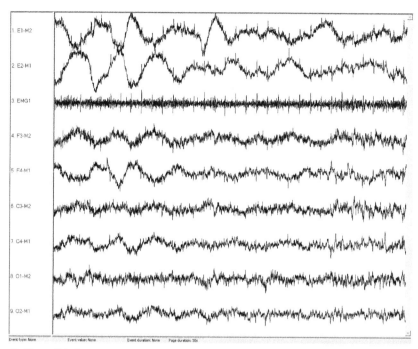

Fig. 2. Stage N1 sleep.

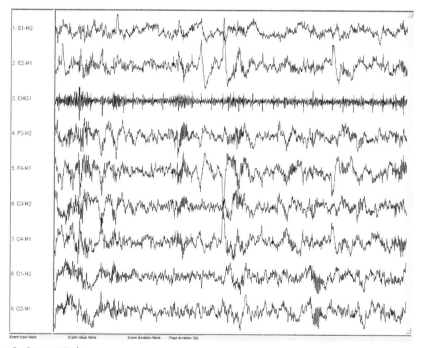

Fig. 3. Stage N2 sleep.

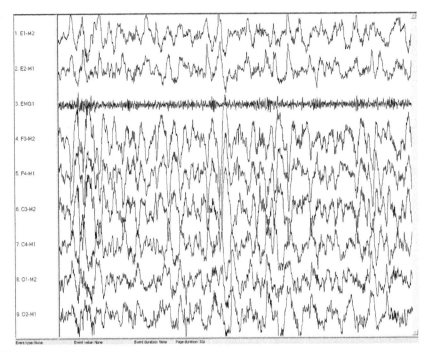

Fig. 4. Stage N3 sleep.

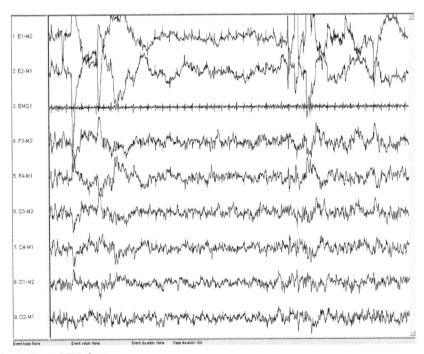

Fig. 5. Stage REM sleep.

IDENTIFYING ABNORMAL SLEEP-RELATED EVENTS

PSG is indicated for the diagnosis of sleep-related breathing disorders (SRBD) and periodic limb movements during sleep (PLMS), titration of positive airway pressure therapy for SRBDs, and evaluation of hypersomnia, atypical parasomnias, and suspected nighttime seizures.

The recommended monitor for identifying apneas is the oronasal thermal sensor. An apnea is defined as a decrease in peak thermal sensor amplitude by at least 90% of baseline for 10 seconds or more and can be obstructive (inspiratory effort is present throughout the entire event) (**Fig. 6**), central (inspiratory effort is absent throughout the entire event) (**Fig. 7**), or mixed (central event followed by an obstructive event) (**Fig. 8**). Measuring respiratory effort using either esophageal manometry or inductance plethysmography is, therefore, important because it can help distinguish between obstructive, central, and mixed apneas. A nasal air pressure transducer and end-tidal carbon dioxide (CO_2) or summed calibrated inductance plethysmography can also be used to detect apneas in adults and children, respectively.

The nasal air pressure transducer is the recommended technique for identifying hypopneas, but inductance plethysmography or oronasal thermal sensors are also useful. Hypopnea is characterized by a decrease in nasal pressure by at least 30% of baseline for a duration of 10 seconds or more and accompanied by at least 4% oxygen desaturation (**Fig. 9**). Oxygen saturation is monitored using pulse oximetry, and alveolar hypoventilation can be inferred from end-tidal or transcutaneous CO_2.

EMG placed over the lower extremities (anterior tibialis) is used to detect PLMS. Additional EMG electrodes can be attached to the upper extremities (extensor digitorum communis) to help identify REM sleep behavior disorder, a type of parasomnia.

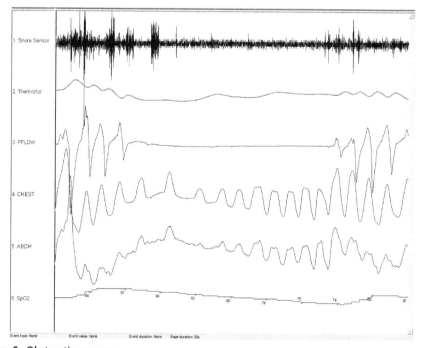

Fig. 6. Obstructive apnea.

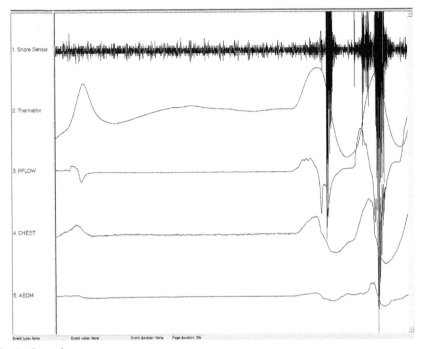

Fig. 7. Central apnea.

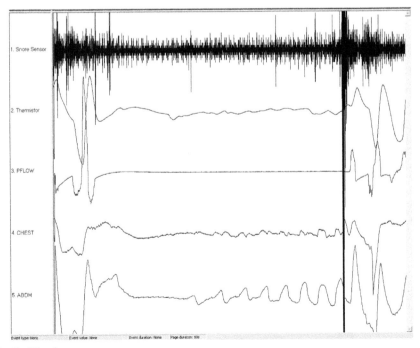

Fig. 8. Mixed apnea.

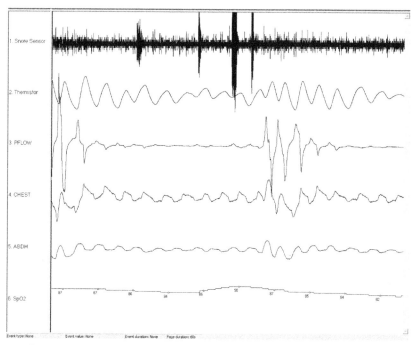

Fig. 9. Obstructive hypopnea.

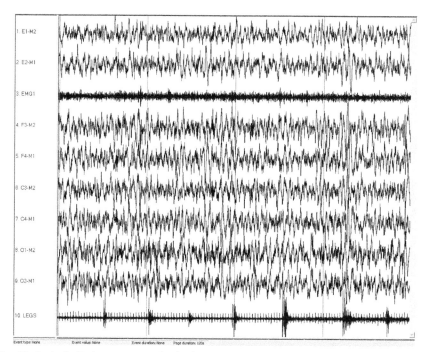

Fig. 10. Periodic limb movements in the leg EMG tracing.

PLMS are scored if there are 4 or more consecutive leg movements, each 0.5 to 10.0 seconds in duration and occurring 5 to 90 seconds between movements (**Fig. 10**).

SUMMARY

Sleep and waking are generated and regulated by specific, but interrelated, neural processes. Wake-promoting systems activate thalamocortical systems, and coordinated removal of arousal systems leads to hyperpolarization of thalamocortical neurons (wake-sleep switch). Activation of GABA and pontine cholinergic neurons promote sleep and generate REM sleep, respectively. Genetically determined circadian rhythms also influence the timing and quality of wakefulness and sleep. Widespread changes in physiologic processes occur during sleep, and these may influence the presentation as well as the severity of specific medical disorders.

REFERENCES

1. Borbely AA. A two process model of sleep regulation. Hum Neurobiol 1982;1: 195–204.
2. Folkard S, Akerstedt T. A three-process model of the regulation of alertness-sleepiness. In: Broughton RJ, Ogilvie R, editors. Sleep, arousal and performance: problems and promises. Boston: Birkhauser; 1992. p. 11–26.
3. Zeitzer JM. Neurochemistry of sleep. In: Amlaner CJ, Fuller PM, editors. Basics of sleep guide. 2nd edition. Westchester (IL): Sleep Research Society; 2009. p. 63–8.
4. Fuller PM, Lu J. Neurobiology of sleep. In: Amlaner CJ, Fuller PM, editors. Basics of sleep guide. 2nd edition. Westchester (IL): Sleep Research Society; 2009. p. 53–62.
5. Morgenthaler TI, Kapur VK, Brown T, et al. Practice parameters for the treatment of narcolepsy and other hypersomnias of central origin. Sleep 2007;30:1705–11.
6. Krystal A. A compendium of placebo-controlled trials of the risks/benefits of pharmacological treatments for insomnia: the empirical basis for U.S. clinical practice. Sleep Med Rev 2009;4:265–74.
7. Sheer FA, Wright KP Jr, Kronauer RE, et al. Plasticity of the intrinsic period of the human circadian timing system. PLoS One 2007;2:e721.
8. Reppert SM, Weaver DR. Circadian regulation of sleep in mammals: role of the suprachiasmatic nucleus. Brain Res Brain Res Rev 2005;49:429–54.
9. Somers VK, Dyken ME, Mark AL, et al. Sympathetic-nerve activity during sleep in normal subjects. N Engl J Med 1993;328:303–7.
10. Orem J, Kubin L. Respiratory physiology: central neural control. In: Kryger MH, Roth T, Dement WC, editors. Principles and practice of sleep medicine. 4th edition. Philadelphia: Elsevier; 2005. p. 213–23.
11. Kario K, Schwartz JE, Pickering TG. Ambulatory physical activity as a determinant of diurnal blood pressure variation. Hypertension 1999;34:685–91.
12. Leproult R, Spiegel K, Van Cauter E. Sleep and endocrinology. In: Amlaner CJ, Fuller PM, editors. Basics of sleep guide. 2nd edition. Westchester (IL): Sleep Research Society; 2009. p. 157–67.
13. Bach V, Telliez F, Libert JP. The interaction between sleep and thermoregulation in adults and neonates. Sleep Med Rev 2002;6:481–92.
14. Opp MR. Cytokines and sleep. Sleep Med Rev 2005;9:355–64.
15. American Academy of Sleep Medicine. The international classification of sleep disorders, second edition: diagnostic and coding manual. Westchester (IL): American Academy of Sleep Medicine; 2005.

Screening and Comprehensive Evaluation for Sleep Related Breathing Disorders

Dennis R. Bailey, DDS[a,b,]*, Ronald Attanasio, DDS, MSEd, MS[c]

KEYWORDS

- Oral evaluation • Nasal airway • Dentist • Oral Health
- Screening

The dentist is well positioned to screen for patients at risk for a sleep disorder and, when adequately trained, can treat those diagnosed with sleep apnea using an oral appliance. This treatment requires some degree of training to be able to recognize the symptoms related to the more common sleep disorders. The dentist must determine if the patient is at risk for a sleep disorder through the use of screening questionnaires, reviewing the health history, and additional questioning of the patient.

The role of the dentist is expanding rapidly as it relates to having a role in the management of medical conditions, particularly because patients' overall health may be impacted by their oral health. This relationship is becoming most apparent in the literature as it relates to the increased risk for cardiovascular disease in individuals with periodontal disease.[1] A direct link has been recognized that compels practicing dentists to be more proactive in managing the periodontal disease process for dental and medical reasons.

Studies have shown that practicing dentists with some knowledge of sleep disorders are just as likely to recognize a patient who may have a sleep disorder as a physician.[2] The average dentist along with the dental hygienist may see just as many patients on a daily basis as a family practitioner or an internist. When a physician is properly trained to evaluate for a sleep disorder or to obtain a sleep history, the possibility of uncovering one has been shown to be more likely.[3] The same can be said for the dentist who sees patients on a regular basis.

[a] Orofacial Pain and Dental Sleep Medicine, Dental Sleep Medicine Mini-Residency, UCLA School of Dentistry, 10833 Le Conte Avenue, CHS-Box 951668, Los Angeles, CA 90095, USA
[b] Private Practice, Denver, CO, USA
[c] University of Nebraska College of Dentistry, Lincoln, NE 68583, USA
* Corresponding author. 8400 East Prentice Avenue, Suite 804, Greenwood Village, CO 80111.
E-mail address: RMC4E@aol.com

Dent Clin N Am 56 (2012) 331–342
doi:10.1016/j.cden.2012.01.007
0011-8532/12/$ – see front matter © 2012 Elsevier Inc. All rights reserved.

SCREENING BY THE DENTIST

The first step for the dentist is to be able to screen for a sleep disorder, most often sleep apnea. This screening can be performed with the addition of very basic and simple questions to an existing health questionnaire, or the dental office can use the Epworth Sleepiness Scale (ESS). The ESS is a questionnaire commonly used in sleep medicine to evaluate a patient's risk for daytime sleepiness and other risk factors. A more basic set of four questions, represented by the acronym *STOP*, can be easily added to an already existing form.[4] Positive responses to two or more of the questions represent an increased risk for sleep apnea. Recently this has been expanded to the STOP-BANG questionnaire. These added four questions seem to be more definitive for determining risk for sleep apnea (**Table 1**). A recent study determined that the use of these questions was able to highly predict sleep apnea.[5] The study showed that a score of three or less had a low probability of predicting sleep apnea. However, the probability increased with a score of between three and five. If the score was greater than five, then the patient had a larger risk for having a severe sleep apnea. Essentially, if the score is zero to three, other risk factors must be considered. If the score is five or greater, the risk for severe sleep apnea increases even more. For example, if the score is eight, the probability for severe sleep apnea is nearly 82%.

Five basic questions may be easily added to those that dentists currently use when taking a health history, and may help identify the presence of a sleep disorder:

1. Do you have difficulty falling asleep or staying asleep?
2. Do you snore?
3. Are you frequently tired during the day?
4. Are you aware or have you been told that you stop breathing during sleep?
5. Is your sleep unrefreshing?

Positive responses to these questions would indicate that further evaluation is needed. At this point patients should complete the ESS and STOP-BANG questionnaires. In the presence of positive responses, patients should then be referred to their physician or a sleep medicine specialist who can further evaluate their needs.

A major concern is that the dentist may not be adequately aware or trained in sleep medicine to recognize the importance of this situation. Therefore, through asking basic questions, the possible risk may be uncovered so that the patient's situation can be adequately addressed. Unfortunately, most dentists are not well versed in sleep medicine and related disorders. One study found that a large number of dentists were not able to recognize when a patient might be at risk for sleep apnea.[6] However, this is slowly changing as more articles are appearing in professional journals read by dentists, continuing education courses are being presented in dental schools, and, in

Table 1 The STOP-BANG questionnaire	
First Four Questions	**Four Additional Questions**
S: snore loudly	B: body mass index >28
T: feel tired during the day	A: age >50 years
O: observed/witnessed to have stopped breathing	N: neck size: male, ≥17 in; female, ≥16 in
P: high blood pressure	G: gender; are you a male
Yes to two or more above: at risk for sleep apnea	Add one or more from above: increased risk for moderate to severe sleep apnea

some cases, the predoctoral curriculum is beginning to include information about sleep and sleep disorders in some of the coursework.

Clinical Recognition of Risk for a Sleep-Related Breathing Disorder

Aside from gathering information from the health history, dentists using the ESS or STOP-BANG questionnaire must be acquainted with the clinical observations seen on a daily basis that may indicate the risk for sleep apnea. Without adequate training or awareness, the dentist may not connect these frequent findings with the risk for a sleep-related breathing disorder (sleep apnea). Recognition of these clinical findings should lead to a more detailed discussion about risk for sleep apnea, or may even lead to a more extensive examination of the oropharyngeal area in addition to the oral cavity.

The best way for those who provide oral health care, including the dental hygienist, to recognize these findings is to become familiar with the conditions that may be encountered and what these may indicate. A simplified way of correlating the clinical observations with how they may indicate a risk for sleep apnea is presented in **Table 2**.

Other sleep disorders commonly seen in practice may be uncovered by the dentist, such as in patients who present with orofacial pain or complaints of headaches who may be at risk for insomnia. Dentists will frequently treat patients for bruxism with various types of splints or appliances. The occurrence of bruxism may indicate an increased risk for restless legs syndrome or periodic limb movement disorder.[7] If a patient is found to be at risk for a sleep disorder, it is important for yhe dentist to know what additional questions to ask to confirm this and how to properly refer the patient for more definitive care.

The Detailed Evaluation

When the dentist is actively involved in the management of a patient with sleep apnea using an oral appliance, the need for a more detailed evaluation is essential. This evaluation would be adjunctive to the routine clinical data that may already exist if that individual is currently a patient of record. Regardless, the dentist must have some format for evaluating the patient to record data relevant to the treatment.

A more detailed evaluation is designed to assess a wide variety of factors in the oral cavity, head, neck, and airway. These areas may be of specific concern not only dentally but also as they relate to the oropharynx and nasal airway, because they may impact the proposed use of an oral appliance. This examination will not only evaluate the past history but also review the patient's medical status, and should involve a review of the findings from the sleep study.

Medical history and chief complaints

The process of taking a patient's medical history and chief complaints would collect information in a question-and-answer format about the patient's symptoms and concerns. This evaluation might include questions related to common symptoms of a sleep disorder, such as poor or disturbed sleep, daytime sleepiness or feeling tired, snoring, observed apneas, tooth grinding (bruxism), headaches, acid reflux (gastro-esophageal reflux disease), depression, mood swings or irritability, poor concentration, and low energy levels. This evaluation would summarize the findings from a sleep study if one was performed before this visit, and might investigate the use of continuous positive airway pressure (CPAP) along with the patient's experience related to its use.

Review of the medical history

A review of the medical history would consider the patient's current medical status along with any medications being taken. At this time, the possible health consequences

Table 2
Clinical findings that may indicate a risk for sleep-related breathing disorders

Clinical Observation	Potential Relationship
Tongue	
Coated	At risk for gastroesophageal reflux disease or mouth-breathing habit
Enlarged	Increased tongue activity, possible OSA
Scalloping at lateral borders (crenations)	Increased risk for sleep apnea[23]
Obstructs view of oropharynx (Mallampati score)	I and II lower risk for OSA III and IV increased risk for OSA
Teeth and periodontal structures	
Gingival inflammation	Mouth-breather, poor oral hygiene
Gingival bleeding when probed	At risk for periodontal disease
Dry mouth (xerostomia)	Mouth-breather: may be medication-related
Gingival recession	May be at risk for clenching
Tooth wear	May have sleep bruxism
Abfraction (cervical abrasion/wear)	Increased parafunction/clenching
Airway	
Long slopping soft palate	At risk for OSA
Enlarged/swollen/elongated uvula	At risk for OSA/snoring
Red patches on posterior pharyngeal wall	At risk for gastroesophageal reflux disease or allergy
Extraoral	
Chapped lips or cracking at the corners of the mouth	Inability to nose-breathe
Poor lip seal/difficulty maintaining a lip seal	Chronic mouth breather
Mandibular retrognathia	Risk for OSA/snoring
Long face (doliocephalic)	Chronic mouth-breathing habit
Enlarged masseter muscle	Clenching/sleep bruxism
Nose/nasal airway	
Small nostrils (nares)	Difficulty nose breathing
Alar rim collapse with forced inspiration	At risk for OSA/sleep-related breathing disorder
Posture of the head/neck	
Forward head posture	Airway compromise and restriction
Loss of lordotic curve	Chronic mouth breather
Posterior rotation of the head	Tendency to mouth-breathe

Abbreviation: OSA, obstructive sleep apnea.

of the sleep disorder, and more specifically sleep apnea, may become evident. Special emphasis should be directed toward headaches, cardiovascular disease, diabetes, asthma, allergy, neurocognitive difficulties, and any medications that are being used to manage these conditions. The patient's blood pressure should also be recorded, which is common in most dental practices.

Evaluation of temporomandibular joints, temporomandibular disorders, orofacial pain

The temporomandibular joints (TMJs) should be evaluated for joint sounds, joint tenderness, or pain, and any dysfunction with mandibular movement. The range of motion of the mandible should also be recorded. Many dentists do not have an adequate background for evaluating these areas, but should become well educated and trained in this process. Any additional orofacial pain complaints other than a temporomandibular dysfunction (TMD) must also be reviewed before any treatment is initiated.

Evaluation of muscle tenderness

Muscle tenderness in the head and neck is often a component of TMD and may be related to bruxism. Travel and Simons[8] found that muscles may have trigger points with the potential to refer pain to a distant location. In the head and neck, the activation of these trigger points may be responsible for complaints of facial pain, headache, sinus pain, TMD, and otalgia. Some of the most commonly encountered muscles and areas of referral are as follows:

- Masseter muscle: this may refer to the maxillary and mandibular molars, the area around the TMJ, the ear, the temples, and the face
- Sternocleidomastoid: this may refer to the forehead, the ear, the face, the top and back of the head, and over the eye. Pain in this muscle may be associated with sleep-disordered breathing because it functions as a secondary muscle in respiration and elevates the rib cage and sternum. This muscle is critical to evaluate in the presence of frontal headaches. It has the potential to refer pain across the midline and is often described as a thigh band around the head
- Temporalis: this may refer to the side of the head and to the maxillary teeth
- Lateral pterygoid: this is often an overlooked muscle and may refer to the face in the area of the zygomatic arch, to the TMJ, and even to the ear.

Dentists should evaluate patients for tenderness involving the muscles of the head and neck, because these may become painful if an oral appliance is used in the future. Whether palpable muscle tenderness is present is important to know in advance so that the possibility of myofascial pain associated with the use of an oral appliance may be anticipated. Measuring the mandibular range of motion first has been recommended, because palpation may aggravate the muscles, thus limiting the movement of the mandible.[9] Often the patient has mostly muscle or myofascial pain that may refer to the TMJ or the surrounding areas, and would then be viewed as TMJ, or *TMD* as it is better known. Poor sleep and TMD are well-known to often coexist.[9]

Dental/oral evaluation

All dentists are comfortable in evaluating the dental and supporting structures of the oral cavity. This part of the evaluation is designed to assess for conditions that may impact use of the oral appliance or may be affected by it. In particular, the dentist must assess for periodontal disease and, more specifically, loose teeth. The presence of dental caries also must be evaluated. If the patient is on medication, concern about xerostomia must also be addressed. Certain oral and dental findings may be present that would limit the success of an oral appliance. These findings might include large mandibular tori, a high palatal vault associated with a narrow maxilla or posterior cross-bite, and teeth that are very short clinically, which may impact the secure retentive fit of the oral appliance.

The tongue also should be evaluated in terms of its position in the mouth at rest relative to the soft palate and the ability to view the oropharynx. This evaluation is referred to as the *Mallampati score* and was revised by Freidman and Tanyeri.[10] This tool uses a scale from I to IV, with I representing a position that allows a full view of the oropharynx and IV representing a position that totally obstructs a full view of oropharynx, soft palate, and uvula (**Table 3**). The more the tongue base obstructs the view of the oropharynx and even the soft palate, the more likely the patient is to be at risk for sleep apnea. One study showed that as the Mallampati score increases, so does the potential risk for obstructive sleep apnea and the potential for an elevation in the apnea-hypopnea index.[11] However, the downward slope of the soft palate should also be viewed, because if the soft palate is extended further into the oropharyngeal region, the Mallampati score may be higher than reflected. A study using videofluoroscopy found that patients with sleep apnea have longer soft palates.[12]

The lingual frenum found at the inferior surface of the tongue at the floor of the mouth should also be evaluated. If the frenum is limiting tongue mobility, the tongue may be more likely to be at a lower position and not rest in the palate as it should, and might cause the tongue base to be farther back into the oropharynx.

Airway evaluation

From the dental perspective, airway evaluation should consider the size of the uvula in terms of its length and mass. The tonsils should be evaluated on a 0 to 4 scale, as is customary in medicine (**Table 4**). As this evaluation is being performed, the presence of the gag reflex also must be considered. Often with sleep-disordered breathing, the gag reflex is lost or significantly diminished.

Cervical spine and postural evaluation

The head posture as it relates to the cervical spine is also important to evaluate. Poor posture, especially as it relates to the head and neck, may be a causative factor as it relates to pain, headache, TMD, and even disturbed sleep. At the same time, poor posture, especially as it relates to the head and cervical spine, may indicate an existing airway problem. During sleep, and even during the time one is awake, the alteration in head position relative to the cervical spine may indicate the presence of airway compromise or difficulty breathing.

On clinical evaluation, several factors may indicate a postural problem associated with an airway issue. Addressing these findings along with the airway problems or the sleep disorder may have a positive impact on the overall treatment. The common findings associated with postural dysfunction that can be assessed on clinical evaluation are as follows:

- Forward head posture: here the head is forward of the shoulders, most often visualized as the ear being forward relative to the height of the shoulder
- Shoulder heights: when viewing the patient from the front, the shoulder heights should be even

Table 3
Description of the Mallampati score

Score	What is Observed with the Tongue at Rest Mouth Wide Open
I	Visualize the soft palate, uvula, tonsils, and the oropharynx
II	Visualize the soft palate, most of the uvula, superior portion of the tonsils, not the oropharynx
III	Can see the soft palate but not the uvula, tonsils, or into the oropharynx
IV	Cannot see the soft palate or any structures below this, can only see the hard palate

Grade	Evaluation of the Tonsillar Size
Table 4 **Assessment of tonsillar size**	
0	Tonsils not visible, most likely have been removed
1	Barely visible, contained within the tonsillar fossa (pillars)
2	Tonsils slightly enlarged, extend beyond the tonsillar fossa (pillars) into the oropharynx
3	Tonsils enlarged, extend approximately half way between the tonsillar fossa and the midline
4	Tonsils very enlarged, extend to the midline, often termed *kissing tonsils*

- Relationship of the occipital area of the skull to the cervical spine (*posterior rotation*): here the head seems to be rotated posteriorly when viewed from the side, and the chin may seem to be tipped up
- Range of motion of the head as it relates to the cervical spine: the head should freely move to the right and left so that the chin is almost over the shoulder. When the head is in flexion the chin should nearly touch the chest, and when in extension the back of the head should be equally rotated to the posterior. All of these movements should be pain-free and not feel tight or restrictive.
- Loss of the lordotic curve: when looking at the patient from the side, the cervical spine should have a slight curve, often referred to as a reverse C shape. If the head is forward, the neck will seem to be straight or even angled forward (forward head posture).

All of these findings can be addressed with physical medicine and a defined exercise program. However, if the airway is compromised or obstructed, the posture of the head as it relates to the cervical spine may be more difficult to manage or correct. In these cases, head position may be compensating for the compromised or obstructed airway.

Abnormal head position, poor posture, the posterior rotation of the occipital area to the first cervical vertebrae, and the loss of the lordotic curve often can be visualized on a lateral head film (cephalometric radiograph). When the head is rotated to the posterior, the chin will often appear up and the occipital area will look compressed and in close relationship to the vertebral process of the first cervical vertebrae. This space is referred to as the *occipital atlas space* (OA space) and will appear compressed. Rocabado[13] described and measured this on cephalometric films and described several measurements that can be used to determine whether the patient has radiographic findings that would suggest postural dysfunction. The OA space is measured from the base of the occipital area to the vertebral process of the first cervical vertebrae. This distance should be 6.5 mm, as should the distance between the first and second vertebral process. When these are compressed so that these measurements are reduced, this indicates that the posture of the cervical spine may be affected by the airway. In addition, the compression of the OA space may compress the greater occipital nerve, which can then lead to headaches and facial pain of cervical origin.

In addition to the cervical spine, the hyoid can also be viewed. As described in other publications, the hyoid position is one definitive observation that indicates an increased risk for sleep apnea.[14] If the hyoid bone is more inferior and posterior and at an increased distance inferior to the border of the mandible, this indicates an increased risk for a sleep-related breathing disorder.[15]

It is also possible that the posterior aspect of the airway may be impacting the airway because of some dysfunction or alteration in the posture of the cervical spine.[16]

Some reports have shown that the posterior aspect of the airway may be pushed inward or that an osteophyte involving the cervical vertebrae may actually impact the posterior aspect of the pharynx.[17]

The Nasal Airway Evaluation

One of the key elements related to successful treatment involves the patient's ability to breathe through the nose. Nasal airway screening or evaluation is not something that is routinely performed before initiating treatment for sleep apnea or snoring. Dentists must become acquainted with the process of screening for a nasal airway problem so they can make an appropriate referral to an otorhinolaryngologist.

Many people have difficulty breathing through the nose, particularly at night, leading to an increased tendency to become mouth-breathers. The resolution of this has become a key factor in CPAP tolerance and effectiveness, and may impact improved oxygen saturation levels during sleep.[18] This condition may be equally important for successful treatment with oral appliances and even surgery, because the nose is viewed as the carburetor of the body. Air flowing through the nose is warmed to body temperature and is humidified to approximately 80%.[19] This process improves the lung's ability to absorb the oxygen in the inspired air. In addition, the nose, and specifically the inferior turbinates, filter the air. Patients who have difficulty breathing through their nose should also be evaluated for allergy.

A questionnaire to determine a patient's subjective assessment of nasal airway problems might be helpful. One that is simple to use and can be combined with the ESS is the Nasal Obstruction Symptom Evaluation (NOSE) scale (**Fig. 1**).[20] The NOSE scale includes five questions and asks the patient to rate their perception of

Nasal Airway / Breathing Assessment
Recently how much have the following
conditions been a concern or problem
(place a mark on the line that
best describes your experience)

Minimal   Severe

Nasal
congestion |————————————————|
stuffiness
obstruction

Difficult to
nose breathe |————————————————|
when sleeping

Difficult to
nose breathe |————————————————|
with exercise
or exertion

Difficult to
nose breathe |————————————————|
in general

Fig. 1. NOSE scale. (*Data from* Stewart MG, Witsell DL, Smith TL, et al. Development and validation of the Nasal Obstruction Symptom Evaluation (NOSE) scale. Otolaryngol Head Neck Surg 2004;130:157–63.)

nasal airway problems over the past month based on a scale of 0 to 4 (ranging from no problem to a severe problem). It then uses a visual analog scale to determine the patient's perception of how difficult it is on average to breathe through the nose.

Dentists must be familiar with how to perform a cursory nasal airway evaluation. If nasal airway obstruction or dysfunction seems to be present, then the patient should be referred for more definitive treatment. The ultimate goal is to improve the chances that the patient is nose-breathing at night, thus lessening mouth-breathing, improving sleep, and even reducing the severity of the obstructive sleep apnea.[21]

Nasal airway anatomy

Dentists or anyone screening for nasal airway problems should be acquainted with the following important areas of the nose (**Fig. 2**):

- The alar rim: the outer area of the nose that is occasionally referred to as the *external nasal valve*. This outer area surrounds the lateral aspect of the nose and helps form the nares (nostril).
- The turbinates: although three paired turbinates are present, the main concern is specifically with the inferior turbinates, because these filter the air. The middle and superior turbinates warm and humidify the air. Enlargement of the inferior turbinates may lead to nasal airway obstruction, narrowing of the nasal valve, and difficulty breathing. The result may be obvious in more of a tendency to mouth breathe.
- The nasal septum: divides the nose into two compartments or sides. Deviation of this can lead to airway obstruction.
- The columella: an area at the midline of the nose located between the two nostrils that is evident externally.
- The nasal valve: an area that is typically viewed as long and narrow, is just inside the nose, and is formed medially by the nasal septum and laterally by the inferior turbinates. Narrowing of this area leads to increased nasal airway resistance and may promote more of a mouth-breathing habit.

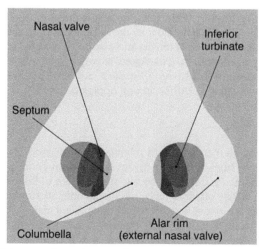

Fig. 2. Anatomy of the nose from the outside area that is important to the dentist release. (*Courtesy of* Dennis R. Bailey, DDS.)

Nasal airway testing

The first nasal airway test is to determine whether the alar rims collapse during forced inspiration through the nose. If the alar rims collapse during nasal inspiration, this may indicate a risk for increased nasal airway resistance. The second test is to determine whether nasal airway dilation improves the patient's ability to nose breath. This test is referred to as the *Cottle test*, and performed simply by placing the fingers at the corners of the nose lateral to the alar rims and gently placing an outward (lateral) force. If results are positive, then some type of nasal airway dilation may be helpful. Ultimately surgery may also prove beneficial.

Treatment options

A variety of noninvasive treatment options can be used if any of the testing is positive for nasal airway compromise:

- Nasal dilation using nasal dilator strips or other types of nasal dilators. Currently several nasal dilators are available that can be inserted into the nose to prevent alar rim collapse and improve the caliber of the nasal valve. These have been shown to also decrease nasal airway resistance.[22]
- Nasal irrigation with a saline and sodium bicarbonate mixture can be helpful with the reduction of inflammation and the removal of foreign material that contributes to nasal airway obstruction. Several over-the-counter products are available or patients may chose to make their own.
- Nasal sprays can be prescribed to reduce inflammation. Some of these sprays are useful for allergies that may be affecting the nasal airway, and typically are antihistamine sprays or nasal steroids.

Improvement of the nasal airway alone may have an impact on the ability to breathe more comfortably. Through reducing the nasal airway resistance, inspiratory drive can also be reduced, which may reduce snoring and improve apnea.

Patients who have significant nasal airway obstruction should be referred to an otorhinolaryngologist for a more detailed evaluation, and nasal endoscopy may be indicated to more completely evaluate the nasal airway, nasopharynx, and vocal chords; look for nasal polyps; and evaluate other related structures, including the tonsils and adenoids. After this testing, more aggressive treatment may be deemed necessary, including surgery or long-term medication use.

Nasal airway surgery that ultimately may prove beneficial include septoplasty, inferior turbinate reduction, removal of tonsils and adenoids, removal of polyps, and other upper airway surgical procedures. Often nasal airway surgery alone is not found to be curative for sleep-related breathing disorders but can be helpful in improving outcomes for patients using CPAP or an oral appliance.

SUMMARY

The dentist can assume many different roles in the evaluation of patients for sleep-disordered breathing, from screening to active involvement in management, often using an oral appliance. As dentists become more aware of the health-related implications of conditions they observe daily, additional education and training regarding sleep disorders will be necessary for optimum patient care. The first step is to become aware of conditions involving the head and neck that may indicate an increased level of risk. Increased understanding of findings in the medical history and of the importance of the nasal airway will lead to improved quality of life for patients.

REFERENCES

1. Demmer RT, Desvarieux M. Periodontal infections and cardiovascular disease. JADA 2006;137(Special Suppl):145–205.
2. Schwarting S, Netzer NC. Sleep apnea for the dentist: political means and practical performance. Presented at Sleep Utah 2006 (0556), Annual Meeting of the APSS. Salt Lake City (UT), June 2006.
3. Haponik EF, Frye AW, Richards B, et al. Sleep history is neglected diagnostic information. J Gen Intern Med 1996;11:759–61.
4. Chung F, Yegneswaran B, Liao P, et al. STOP questionnaire. Anesthesiology 2008;108:812–21.
5. Silva GE, Vana KD, Goodwin JL, et al. Identification of patients with sleep disordered breathing: comparing the four-variable screening tool, STOP, STOP-Bang, and Epworth Sleepiness Scales. J Clin Sleep Med 2011;7(5):467–72.
6. Bian H. Knowledge, opinions, and clinical experience of general practice dentists toward obstructive sleep apnea and oral appliances. Sleep Breath 2004;8(2): 85–90.
7. Lavigne GJ, Montplaisir JY. Restless legs syndrome and sleep bruxism: prevalence and association among Canadians. Sleep 1994;17(8):739–43.
8. Travel JG, Simons DG. Myofascial pain and dysfunction the trigger point manual. Baltimore (MD): Williams and Wilkins; 1983.
9. Wright EF. Manual of temporomandibular disorders. Ames (IA): Blackwell; 2005. p. 27.
10. Freidman M, Tanyeri H, La Rosa M, et al. Clinical predictors of obstructive sleep apnea. Laryngoscope 1999;109:1901–7.
11. Nuckton TJ, Glidden DV, Browner WS, et al. Physical examination: Malampati score as an independent predictor of obstructive sleep apnea. Sleep 2006; 29(7):903–8.
12. Lee CH, Mo J, Kim BJ, et al. Evaluation of soft palate changes using sleep videofluoroscopy in patients with obstructive sleep apnea. Arch Otolaryngol Head Neck Surg 2009;135(2):168–72.
13. Rocabado M. Biomechanical relationship of the cranial, cervical and hyoid regions. J Craniomandibular Pract 1983;1(3):61–6.
14. Hoehema A, Hovinga B, Stegenga B, et al. Craniofacial morphology and obstructive sleep apnea: a cephalometric analysis. J Oral Rehabil 2003;30(7):690–6.
15. Attanasio R, Bailey D. Dental management of sleep disorders. Ames (IA): Wiley-Blackwell; 2010.
16. Finkelstein Y, Wexler D, Horowitz E, et al. Frontal and lateral cephalometry in patients with sleep-disordered breathing. Laryngoscope 2001;111:634–41.
17. Fuerderer S, Eysel-Gosepath K. Retro-pharyngeal obstruction in association with osteophytes of the cervical spine. J Bone Joint Surg Br 2004;86(6):837–40.
18. Pevernagie DA, De Meyer MM, Claeys S. Sleep, breathing and the nose. Sleep Med Rev 2005;9:437–51.
19. Freidman M, Zubair S, Roee L. The role of nasal obstruction and nasal surgery in the pathogenesis and treatment of obstructive sleep apnea and snoring. Curr Opin Otolaryngol Head Neck Surg 2001;9(3):158–61.
20. Stewart MG, Witsell DL, Smith TL, et al. Development and validation of the nasal obstruction symptom evaluation (NOSE) scale. Otolaryngol Head Neck Surg 2004;130:157–63.
21. McLean HA, Urton AM, Driver HS, et al. Effect of treating severe nasal obstruction on the severity of obstructive sleep apnoea. Eur Respir J 2005;25(3):521–7.

22. Peltonen LI, Vento SI, Simola M, et al. Effects of the nasal strip and dilator on nasal breathing: a study with healthy subjects. Rhinology 2004;42(3):122–5.

23. Weiss TM, Atanasov S, Calhoun KH. The association of tongue scalloping with obstructive sleep apnea and related sleep pathology. Otolaryngol Head Neck Surg 2005;133(6):966–71.

Cone Beam Computed Tomography: Craniofacial and Airway Analysis

David C. Hatcher, DDS, MSc[a,b,c],*

KEYWORDS

- Cone beam CT (CBCT) • Volumetric imaging
- Degenerative joint disease • TMJ • Airway • Retroglossal
- Retropalatal • Facial growth

Imaging plays a role in the anatomic assessment of the airway and adjacent structures. Obstructive sleep-disordered breathing (OSDB) is not diagnosed with imaging, but imaging can identify patients with airways who are at risk for obstruction and other anatomic characteristics that may contribute to OSDB. The airway extending from the tip of the nose to the superior end of the trachea can be visualized on conventional computed tomography (CT) and cone beam CT (CBCT) scans. Because these scans also include the jaws, teeth, cranial base, spine, and facial soft tissues, there is an opportunity to evaluate the functional and developmental relationships between these structures. The skeletal support for airway is provided by the cranial base (superiorly), spine (posteriorly), nasal septum (anterosuperiorly), jaws, and hyoid bone (anteriorly). The airway valves include the soft palate, tongue, and epiglottis (**Fig. 1**). Airway obstructions or encroachments are of interest because they increase airway resistance that may contribute to OSDB; therefore, visualization and calculation of the airway dimensions are important. Common airway encroachments include turbinates, adenoids, long soft palate, large tongue, and pharyngeal and lingual tonsils. Less common airway encroachments include polyps and tumors.

This article discusses the use of 3-dimensional (3D) imaging (CBCT) to evaluate the airway and selected regional anatomic variables that may contribute to OSDB. Optimal treatment outcomes begin with a complete and accurate diagnosis. Imaging may assist in delineating attributes that contribute to OSDB in patients who do not have a phenotype (such as high body mass index) that is routinely associated with OSDB.

This article originally appeared in *Sleep Medicine Clinics, Volume 5, Number 1, 2010.*
[a] University of Southern Nevada, 11 Sunset Way, Henderson, NV 89014, USA
[b] Arthur A. Dugoni School of Dentistry, 2155 Webster Street, San Francisco, CA 94115, USA
[c] Private Practice, Diagnostic Digital Imaging, 99 Scripps Drive, #101, Sacramento, CA 95825, USA
* University of Southern Nevada, 11 Sunset Way, Henderson, NV 89014.
E-mail address: David@ddicenters.com

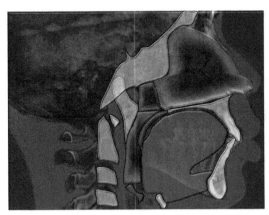

Fig. 1. Airway zones that are visible using CBCT (*blue and green*). These zones extend from the nasal tip to the epiglottis and are divided in the nasal, nasopharyngeal, and oral airways. The airway is supported posteriorly by the spine; superiorly by the cranial base; and anteriorly by the maxilla, mandible, and hyoid (*white*). The mobile elements associated with the airway include the tongue, soft palate, and epiglottis (*red*).

CBCT AND IMAGE ANALYSIS

Technological advances in computing power, sensor technology, and reconstruction algorithms have merged and resulted in the introduction of a CBCT (also known as volumetric imaging). Volumetric imaging is synonymous with 3D imaging because the information has depth in addition to height and width. The 3D imaging domain includes radiograph (CT and CBCT) and magnetic resonance imaging technologies. The 2 principal differences that distinguish CBCT from traditional CT are the type of imaging source-detector complex and the method of data acquisition. The radiograph source for CT is a high-photon, output rotating anode generator, whereas for CBCT it can be a low-energy fixed anode tube similar to that used in dental panoramic machines. CT uses a fan-shaped x-ray beam from its source to acquire images and records data on solid-state image detectors that are arranged in a 360° array around the patient. CBCT technology uses a cone-shaped x-ray beam with a special image intensifier and a solid-state sensor or an amorphous silicon plate for capturing the image.

Conventional medical CT devices image patients in a series of axial plane slices that are captured either as individual stacked slices or using a continuous spiral motion over the axial plane. Conversely, CBCT presently uses one rotation sweep of the patient similar to that used for panoramic radiography. Image data can be collected for either a complete dental/maxillofacial volume or a limited regional area of interest. Scan times for these vary from 8 to 40 seconds for the complete volume. CBCT has a significantly lower radiation burden than a comparable scan using a conventional CT. CBCT has a favorable risk/benefit ratio for many craniofacial applications, including imaging of the airway and associated craniofacial structures.

ANATOMIC ACCURACY

An ideal imaging goal is to accurately represent the anatomy as it exists in nature, that is, the anatomic truth. The projection geometry associated with 2D techniques does not produce accurate anatomic images. 3D digital techniques using back projection algorithms create the opportunity to produce anatomically accurate images.

Current 3D imaging techniques allow an anatomically accurate capture of the surface and subsurface structures.[1–4] One measure of image quality is the ability to detect small anatomic features. The variables that have significant influence on the quality of a CBCT include voxel size (smallest element in a 3D digital image), dynamic range (number of gray levels), signal, and noise. In general, the best quality image is composed of small voxels, large number of gray levels, high signal, and low noise. CBCT voxels are isotropic (equal size in all dimensions x, y, and z) and range in size from 0.1 to 0.4 mm. The captured field of view (FOV) can be scaled to match the regions of interest (ROIs). The ROI can include the entire craniofacial region or a selected subsection of the craniofacial anatomy. The display of the captured FOV or subset of image data can be viewed from any angle using various display techniques (**Fig. 2**). For example, the entire craniofacial skeleton may be captured using a CBCT scan, but using software tools, an ROI (such as the airway) may be selected, displayed, and analyzed. Several software companies have developed application-specific display and analysis software that result in the measurement (linear, area, volume, angular) of segmented and integrated anatomic structures. Of particular interest is the metric analysis of the airway and the adjacent structures. Specialized software for metric analysis of the airway has been calibrated using orthogonal and oblique airway phantoms, and has been validated for accuracy and precision.[2,3] The convergence of CBCT with the application software is very beneficial in understanding and diagnosing OSDB and its relationship to craniofacial anatomy.

FACIAL GROWTH AND THE AIRWAY

Alterations from the normal pattern of nasal respiration occurring during active growth can affect the development of the craniofacial skeleton in humans and experimental animals.[5–8] Severely reduced nasal airflow may induce compensations that include an inferior mandibular rest position, parting of the lips, increased interocclusal space, lower or more forward tongue position, lower positioning of the hyoid bone, a modal shift from nasal breathing to mouth breathing, anterior extension of the head and neck, increased anterior face height, increase in the mandibular and occlusal plane angles, narrow alar base, narrow maxillary arch, high palatal vault, posterior crossbite, class II occlusion, and clockwise facial growth pattern. These compilations of craniofacial and occlusal traits produce a facial phenotype that has been cited in the orthodontic literature as "adenoidal facies," thus ascribing an etiology and expressing a bias that hypertrophic adenoidal tissues are the cause of an obtunded nasal airflow that results in a specific pattern of craniofacial deformation. However, this facial phenotype may also occur secondary to aberrant mandibular growth. The end result in several craniofacial growth scenarios may be associated with alterations in airway dimensions, airway resistance, and functional airway patency, but the cause-and-effect relationships need to be considered. For example, does an anatomic reduction in airway function cause the craniofacial compensations or does abnormal craniofacial growth result in compromised airway function? The anteroposterior dimensions of the airway have been shown to have a proportional relationship to jaw growth and facial growth pattern.[9] The airway is largest when there is normal mandibular and maxillary growth and when facial growth pattern occurs with a counter-clockwise rotation. Conversely, the airway is smaller with deficient maxillary and mandibular growth and when there is a clockwise facial growth pattern. Because mandibular growth has been linked to condylar growth and degenerative joint disease (DJD, also known as osteoarthritis) affects condylar growth, it is reasonable to postulate that a developmental onset of DJD may limit airway dimensions (**Figs. 3** and **4**).

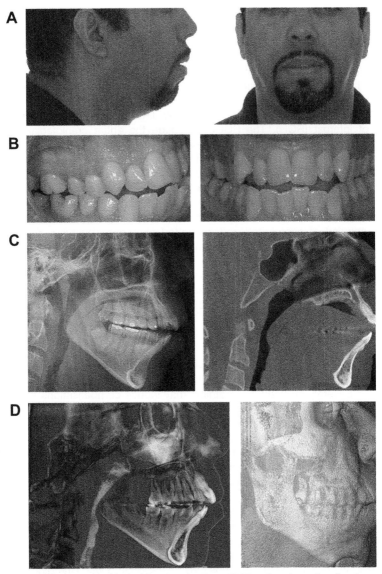

Fig. 2. Craniofacial and airway visualization. Various CBCT and patient visualization options. (*A*, *B*) Convex facial profile, narrow maxilla, anterior open bite, and forward head and neck posture. (*C*) Midsagittal airway (*right image*) and a standard cephalometric image generated from the CBCT volume using specialized software. (*D*) Volume-rendered and shaded surface display image of the head and neck skeleton along with the airway-skin boundaries. (*E*) Analysis of the airway. The midsagittal airway view is mapped (*left image*), and a series of cross-sectional areas (CSAs) of the mapped regions are generated (*right image*). The CSA and distance measurements are calculated and displayed for each of the cross-sectional intervals. The smallest cross-sectional area was identified to be 38.94 mm². (*F*) A reconstructed panoramic projection. The data volume can be reconstructed in any user-defined orthogonal, oblique, or curved plane to match the clinical investigation objective. Note the small condyles and forward posture of the mandible.

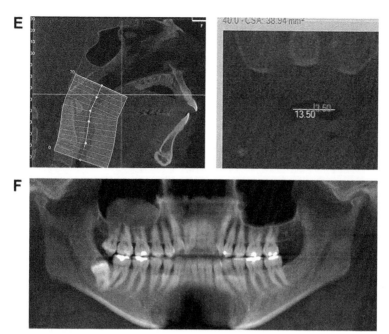

Fig. 2. (*continued*)

Current 3D imaging techniques available for routine imaging provide the opportunity to use a "systems approach" to visualize and evaluate the functional and developmental relationships between proximal craniofacial regions. It has been reported that a developmental insult to the temporomandibular joints (TMJs) may have a regional effect on the growth of the ipsilateral side of the face, including the mandible, maxilla, and base of the skull.[10–18] Similarly, there is a direct relationship between jaw growth and airway development.[9] The notion that there are functional and growth relationships between adjacent anatomic regions creates the desire for a robust method to visualize and analyze them.

MANDIBULAR GROWTH

The mandible forms by using a combination of endochondral and intramembranous processes of bone formation. The condyles do not control growth of the entire mandible, but condylar growth contributes to the process of mandibular growth, primarily the condylar processes and rami, and secondarily the body and alveolar ridges. Mesenchymal cell differentiation into articular cartilage followed by endochondral ossification contributes to the condylar growth. There are several mandibular growth sites (growth fields), including the condyles, alveolar process, rami, body, and coronoid process. These growth sites have genetic potential for growth through mesenchymal cell differentiation and cell division, but the growth can be modulated through external or environmental (epigenetic) factors. These external factors include neighboring growth sites, hormones, tissue stress and strain, and tissue damage. The craniofacial complex generally grows in harmony. Changes occurring in one area of the craniofacial complex induce a response in the adjacent areas. A model proposed by Petrovic and coworkers[12,13] suggests that distant craniofacial changes (such as maxillary growth) are transformed into local (mandibular) growth signals by a complex interplay of muscle adaptation,

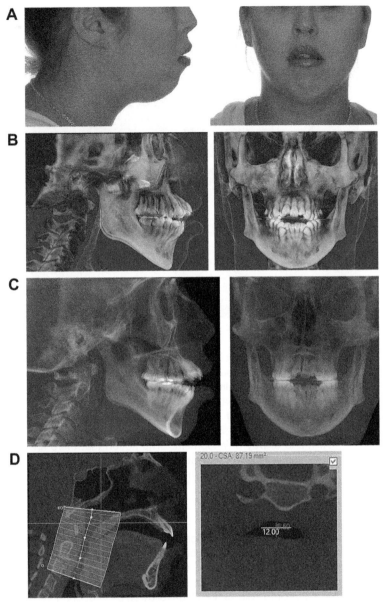

Fig. 3. Temporomandibular joint (TMJ), facial growth, and airway. A craniofacial phenotype that occurs after a developmental onset of TMJ DJD. The DJD limited or arrested the development of the condyles, and this resulted in reduced mandibular growth along with other craniofacial compensations (F). The condyles were located in the anteroinferior regions of their fossa when in habitual occlusion (F). Note the convex facial profile (A–C), the anterior open bite (B–D, E, F), and the forward head and neck posture. The mediolateral development of the maxilla and mandible was reduced (B, C, E), and the tongue was postured down and away from the depth of the palate. There was diffuse narrowing of the airway with the smallest cross-sectional area measuring 87.19 mm^2. The forward posture of the mandible may be a compensation to improve airway patency. Selective muscle recruitment is required to resist the clockwise rotation of the mandible and maintain airway patency.

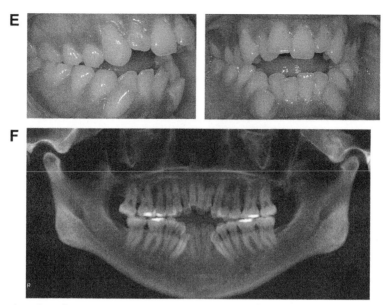

Fig. 3. (*continued*)

neural input, connective tissue response, blood supply, biochemical growth activation, and suppression. Condylar fibrocartilage, during growth, is responsive to growth stimuli from various systemic and local influences. Ideally, condylar growth is modulated to keep pace with facial growth. Fibrocartilage in the adult condyle has an adaptive function to maintain the mandible in its functional role. Reduced adaptive capacity of the fibrocartilage (such as DJD) during growth and development has been shown to limit growth of the ipsilateral half of the mandible. DJD in adulthood that results in significant hard tissue loss may be associated with a change in mandibular posture, occlusion, and condyle/fossa spatial relationships.

DEGENERATIVE JOINT DISEASE

DJD (also known as degenerative arthritis, degenerative arthrosis, osteoarthritis, and osteoarthrosis) affects all joints, including the TMJ. There are several factors that can initiate the pathologic and imaging features associated with DJD. These factors create a situation whereby the articular structures can no longer resist the applied forces to the joint. DJD involves the destruction of the hard and soft articular tissues, and occurs when the remodeling capacity of those tissues has been exceeded by the functional demands. Therefore, scenarios that modulate and increase joint loads or diminish the strength or adaptive capacity of the articular tissues are of interest in discovering the pathogenesis of TMJ DJD. The understanding of DJD has significantly evolved during the past 30 years. Until recently, DJD of the TMJ was considered a wear and tear phenomenon that occurred in individuals older than 40 years, as observed in other synovial joints. However, recent investigations and clinical observations have discovered significant differences in the occurrence and behavior of TMJ DJD in comparison with other joints. TMJ DJD has been recognized to have a predilection for women and can be identified at all ages after puberty, and is not limited to individuals older than 40 years. It has been suggested that sex hormones and hormone receptors may play a role in the early age onset and sex predilection of this phenomenon. DJD onset

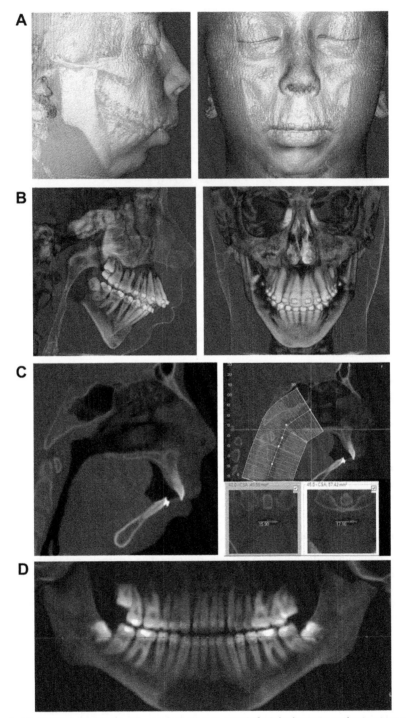

Fig. 4. (*A–D*) TMJ, facial growth, and airway. A craniofacial phenotype that occurs after a developmental onset of TMJ juvenile rheumatoid arthritis (JRA). The regional compensations to the JRA were similar to those observed in **Fig. 3** for DJD. There was a convex facial profile, clockwise facial growth pattern, steep mandibular and occlusal planes, obtuse gonial angles, small mediolateral jaw dimensions, inferior positioning of hyoid bone, anterior open bite, and small airway. The airway dimensions were diffusely narrowed with the smallest cross-sectional area measuring 49.59 mm².

and the associated complaints in women occur from puberty through menopause. The TMJ is a diarthrodial joint like other synovial joints; however, the expression of DJD differs from other joints. Key distinctions between the TMJ anatomy and other synovial joints include the predominance of fibrocartilage in lieu of hyaline cartilage and motion mechanics that include rotation and translation. The TMJ is a loaded joint, and the joint loads or stress concentrations (force/area) may be equal to other load-bearing joints.[18] The functional movement of the condyle over the disk creates a contact force (F) applied in a direction (cos θ) over a distance (d) during a specific time (t) interval. The disk/condyle interactions can be expressed in terms of work (W) or power (P); $W = F \times d \times \cos \theta$ and $P = W/t$.[19–22] Investigators are currently examining the mechanobiology or single-cell biomechanics, that is, how physical forces influence biologic processes in the TMJ.[23–26] Single-cell biomechanics depend on their material properties relative to the surrounding matrix. The TMJ disk cells are a heterogeneous mixture of fibroblasts and fibrochondrocytes. The TMJ disk is a fibrocartilaginous tissue, but it is not a homogeneous tissue. The disk is composed mostly of collagen (type I), proteoglycans (glycosaminoglycan chains that are primarily chondroitin sulfate and dermatan sulfate), and water. The distribution and arrangement of the disk components are not uniform. This disk has been divided into 3 areas or zones: the anterior band, the intermediate zone, and the posterior band. These zones, like anatomic regions, create material property differences, and therefore the single-cell biomechanics between these zones may vary. The anatomic variations between the zones ideally reflect a structural relationship to the functional demands in terms of work and power. The work imparted on the tissues (cells) initiates a mechanotransduction pathway (mechanism by which cells convert a mechanical stimulus into a chemical activity) that results in gene expression. Gene expression initiates several pathways to produce (1) extracellular matrix proteins, (2) matrix metalloproteinases, (3) proinflammatory cytokines, or (4) apoptosis regulators. The extracellular matrix protein

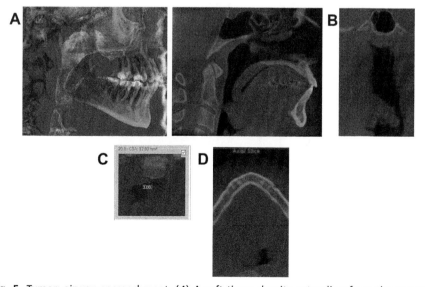

Fig. 5. Tumor; airway encroachment. (*A*) A soft tissue density extending from the tongue base region and encroaching on the airway space. (*B–D*) Soft tissue density extending from the right lateral wall of the oral pharynx. This soft tissue encroachment was determined to be a squamous cell carcinoma that had reduced the cross-sectional area to 87.93 mm².

synthesis creates extracellular matrix and tissue regeneration. The production of matrix metalloproteinases and proinflammatory cytokines results in extracellular matrix degradation. Extracellular matrix degradation and apoptosis are pathways that can result in DJD. The variations in mechanotransduction pathways may be related to the tissue anatomy, tissue quality, and power (work/time). Several variables affect work, including peak forces, force vectors, velocity, and work cycles. The tissues' anatomy and quality will relate to the adaptive capacity of those tissues. Both mechanotransduction and signal transduction by hormones (β-estradiol, relaxin, progesterone) are currently being explored.[27,28] In vivo testing on rabbits using disk explants has demonstrated that increased serum levels of relaxin, β-estradiol and relaxin, and β-estradiol result in the loss of glycosaminoglycans and collagen from fibrocartilaginous sites (ie, TMJ and pubic symphysis) but not from hyaline cartilaginous sites. Relaxin and β-estradiol induced the matrix metalloproteinase expression of collagenase-1 and stromelysin-1. It was also shown that progesterone prevented

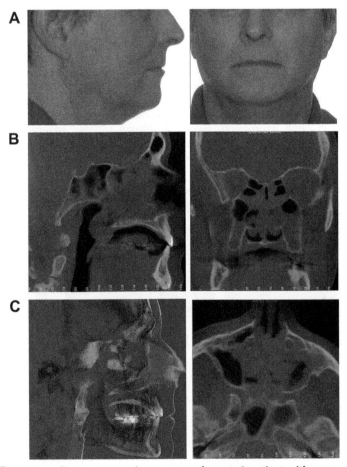

Fig. 6. Inflammatory disease; upper airway encroachment. A patient with severe rhinosinusitis (A). The ostiomeatal units and the nasal fosse were not patent. A polyp was extending into the nasopharynx (B, *left image*). A discontinuity of the airway spaces of the nose and the oral pharynx (C, *left image*) (air shown as white).

the loss of matrix molecules. This hormone-induced, targeted matrix degradation may be the key to the understanding of why TMJ DJD is most commonly seen in women during their reproductive years. There is likely interplay between mechanotransduction and hormonal transduction of matrix degradation proteinases during the onset and progression of DJD.

DJD: IMAGING OBSERVATIONS

Current imaging modalities have revealed several stages associated with DJD that progress along a continuum from normal, failure, repair, and stability.[18] It has been observed that soft tissue changes occur first, and this progresses to the involvement of hard tissues in a small percentage of individuals. It has been proposed that DJD progresses until the functional forces (work and power) are modulated by tissue changes to be within the adaptive capacity of targeted tissues.

AIRWAY

3D imaging is a very efficient method to inspect and identify diffuse narrowing (narrowing disturbed over a large distance) or focal narrowing (encroachments) of the airway. A reduction in airway radius increases the airway resistance as described by Poiseuille's law ($R = 8 nl/pr^4$) where R is resistance, n is viscosity, l is length, and r is

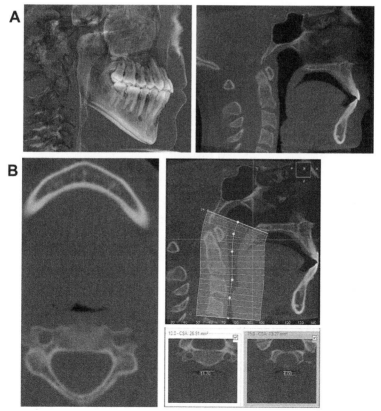

Fig. 7. Lingual tonsils; base of tongue encroachment. (*A, B*) The airway of a patient with large lingual tonsils. The airway at base of the tongue was calculated to be 13.77 mm².

radius. Airflow maintenance requires increased inspiration effort as the resistance to airflow increases as described by Ohm's law ($V = P_{mouth} - P_{alveoli}/R$) where V is flow, P is pressure, and R is resistance. The increased inspiration effort results in a greater differential pressure between the mouth and the alveoli. The airway, an elastic tube, is

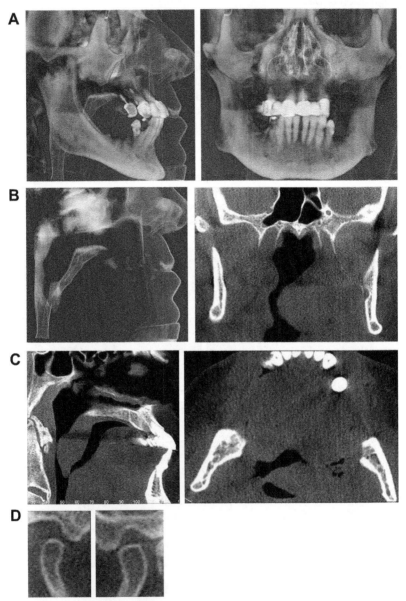

Fig. 8. (A–D) Tumor; upper airway encroachment. This individual was scanned using a CBCT and displayed using multiplanar sections and volume rendering. The condyles were in an acquired anteroinferior position within their fossa. A soft tissue mass was identified, extending from the left lateropharyngeal wall and extending into and enlarging the dimensions of the soft palate. This mass was determined to be a squamous cell carcinoma. The mass had reduced the airway dimensions, and the patient found it necessary to hold the jaw forward to maintain airway patency.

collapsible and is susceptible to the generation of a large pressure gradient between the lung alveoli and mouth. Mobility of the selected airway valves, such as the tongue, nares, soft palate, and epiglottis, may increase under the influence of increased respiratory pressure. Increased resistance in the airway requires a greater inspiratory pressure to maintain airflow predisposing to airway collapse.

Multivariate analysis shows both retroglossal ($P = .027$) and retropalatal spaces ($P = .0036$) to be predictive of respiratory disturbance index. Li and colleagues[29] have also demonstrated a relationship between the airway area and the likelihood of obstructive sleep apnea (OSA). There is a high probability of severe OSA if the airway area is less than 52 mm^2, an intermediate probability if the airway is between 52 to 110 mm^2, and a low probability if the airway is greater than 110 mm^2.[30–32] Lowe and colleagues[30] demonstrated that most constrictions occur in the oropharynx with a mean airway volume of 13.89 ± 5.33 cm^3. Barkdull and colleagues[33,34] demonstrated a correlation between the retro-lingual cross-sectional airway and OSA when this area was less than 4% of the cross-sectional area of the cervicomandibular ring. Encroachments that increase resistance can occur anywhere along the length of the airway and include rhinitis, deviated septum, polyps, tonsils, adenoids, and tumors (see **Fig. 4; Figs. 5–8**).

SUMMARY

Incorporation of 3D imaging into daily practice will allow practitioners to readily evaluate and screen patients for phenotypes associated with OSDB. This is particularly important in the adolescent population where many already seek orthodontic treatment for dentofacial deformities associated with OSDB.

The introduction and availability of CBCT has created the opportunity to serially examine individuals and acquire accurate 3D anatomic information. The "systems approach" of observing and testing the interactions and influence that adjacent regions have on each other will be a key to the understanding of the biomechanical influences on craniofacial form and the role they play in OSDB.

REFERENCES

1. Stratemann S, Huang J, Makik K, et al. Comparison of cone beam computed tomography imaging with physical measures. Dentomaxillofac Radiol 2008; 37(2):80–93.
2. Schendel SA, Hatcher D. CBCT semiautomated 3D airway analysis. J Oral Maxillofac Surg 2010. [Epub ahead of print].
3. Aboudara C, Nielsen I, Huang JC, et al. Comparison of airway space with conventional lateral head films and 3-dimensional reconstruction from cone-beam computed tomography. Am J Orthod Dentofacial Orthop 2009;135(4):468–79.
4. Aboudara CA, Hatcher D, Neilsen IL, et al. A three-dimensional evaluation of the upper airway in adolescents. Orthod Craniofac Res 2003;6(Suppl 1):173–5.
5. Woodside D, Linder-Aronson S, Ludstrom A, et al. Mandibular and maxillary growth after changed mode of breathing. Am J Orthod Dentofacial Orthop 1991;100:1–18.
6. Yamada T, Tanne K, Miyamoto K, et al. Influences of nasal respiratory obstruction on craniofacial growth in young *Macaca fuscata* monkey. Am J Orthod Dentofacial Orthop 1997;11:38–43.
7. Solow B, Siersback-Nielsen S, Greve E. Airway adequacy, head posture, and craniofacial morphology. Am J Orthod 1984;86:214–23.

8. Vargervik K, Miller A, Chierici G, et al. Morphologic response to changes in neuro-muscular patterns experimentally induced by altered modes of respiration. Am J Orthod 1984;85:115–24.

9. Stratemann S. 3D craniofacial imaging: airway and craniofacial morphology [Unpublished MSc thesis], Department of Growth and Development. University of California San Francisco; 2005.

10. Legrell PE, Isberg A. Mandibular length and midline asymmetry after experimentally induced temporomandibular joint disk displacement in rabbits. Am J Orthod Dentofacial Orthop 1999;115(3):247–53.

11. Legrell PE, Isberg A. Mandibular height asymmetry following experimentally induced temporomandibular joint disk displacement in rabbits. Oral Surg Oral Med Oral Pathol Oral Radiol Endod 1998;86(3):280–3.

12. Stutzmann JJ, Patrovic AG. Role of the lateral pterygoid muscle and menisco temporomandibular frenum in spontaneous growth of the mandible and in growth stimulated by the postural hyperpropulsor. Am J Orthod Dentofac Orthop 1990; 97:381–92.

13. Petrovic AG. Heritage paper. Auxologic categorization and chronobiologic specific for the choice of appropriate orthodontic treatment. Am J Orthod Dentofac Orthop 1994;105(2):192–205.

14. Nebbe B, Major PW. Prevalence of TMJ disc displacement in a pre-orthodontic adolescent sample. Angle Orthod 2000;70(6):454–63.

15. Flores-Mir C, Akbarimaned L, Nebbe B, et al. Longitudinal study on TMJ disk status and its effect on mandibular growth. J Orthod 2007;34(3):194–9.

16. Flores-Mir C, Nebbe B, Heo G, et al. Longitudinal study of temporomandibular joint disc status and craniofacial growth. Am J Orthod Dentofacial Orthop 2007;131(5):575–6.

17. Nebbe B, Major PW, Prassad N. Female adolescent facial pattern associated with TMJ disk displacement and reduction in disk length: part I. Am J Orthod Dentofacial Orthop 1999;116(2):168–76.

18. Hatcher DC, McEvoy SP, Mah RT, et al. Distribution of local and general stresses in the stomatognathic system. In: McNeill C, editor. Science and practice of occlusion. Chicago: Quintessence Publishing Co; 1997. p. 259–72.

19. Mah RT, McEvoy SP, Hatcher DC, et al. Engineering principles and modeling strategies. In: McNeill C, editor. Science and practice of occlusion. Chicago: Quintessence Publishing Co; 1997. p. 153–64.

20. Gallo LM, Chiaravolloti G, Iwaskai LR, et al. Mechanical work during stress field translation in the human TMJ. J Dent Res 2006;85(11):1006–10.

21. Nickel JC, Iwasaki LR, Beatty MW, et al. Static and dynamic loading effects on temporomandibular joint disc tractional forces. J Dent Res 2006;85(9): 809–13.

22. Nickel JC, Iwaskai LR, Beatty MW, et al. Laboratory stresses and tractional forces on the TMJ disc surface. J Dent Res 2004;83(8):650–4.

23. Lammi M. Current perspective on cartilage and chondrocyte mechanobiology. Biorheology 2004;41:593–6.

24. Turner CH. Biomechanical aspects of bone formation. In: Bronner F, Farach-Carson MC, editors. Bone formation. London: Springer Press; 2004. p. 79–105.

25. Carter DR, Beaupré GS, Wong M, et al. The mechanobiology of articular cartilage development and degeneration. Clin Orthop Relat Res 2004;(Suppl 427): S69–77.

26. Huang H, Kamm RD, Lee RT, et al. Cell mechanics and mechanotransduction: pathways, probes, and physiology. Am J Physiol Cell Physiol 2004;287:C1–11.

27. Hashem G, Zhang Q, Hayami T, et al. Relaxin and beta-estradiol modulate targeted matrix degradation in specific synovial joint fibrocartilages: progesterone prevents matrix loss. Arthritis Res Ther 2006;8(4):R98.

28. Naqvi T, Duong T, Hashem G, et al. Relaxin's induction of metalloproteinases is associated with loss of collagen and glycosaminoglycans in synovial joint fibrocartilaginous explants. Arthritis Res Ther 2005;7(1):R1–11.

29. Li HY, Chen NH, Wang CR, et al. Use of 3-dimensional computed tomography scan to evaluate upper airway patency for patients undergoing sleep-disordered breathing surgery. Otolaryngol Head Neck Surg 2003;1294:336–42.

30. Lowe AA, Gionhaku N, Takeuchi K, et al. Three-dimensional CT reconstructions of tongue and airway in adult subjects with obstructive sleep apnea. Am J Orthod Dentofacial Orthop 1986;90(5):364–74.

31. Avrahami E, Englender M. Relation between CT axial cross-sectional area of the oropharynx and obstructive sleep apnea syndrome in adults. AJNR Am J Neuroradiol 1995;16(1):135–40.

32. Ogawa T, Enciso R, Shintaku WH, et al. Evaluation of cross-section airway configuration of obstructive sleep apnea. Oral Surg Oral Med Oral Pathol Oral Radiol Endod 2007;103(1):102–8.

33. Chen NH, Li KK, Li SY, et al. Airway assessment by volumetric computed tomography in snorers and subjects with obstructive sleep apnea in a Far-East Asian population (Chinese). Laryngoscope 2002;112(4):721–6.

34. Barkdull GC, Kohl CA, Patel M, et al. Computed tomography imaging of patients with obstructive sleep apnea. Laryngoscope 2008;118:1486–92.

Sleep Study—What the Dentist Needs to Know

John F. Trapp, MD*, T. Troy Stentz, BA, RPSGT

KEYWORDS

- Sleep study • Polysomnogram interpretation
- Sleep related breathing disorder

The intent of this article is to familiarize dental professionals with the polysomnogram (PSG). Through a better understanding of the PSG as a diagnostic tool, dental professionals are able to provide a more comprehensive assessment of individual patients who present with a sleep disorder complaint, including sleep-related breathing disorders (SRBDs).

The initial assessment of patients with a sleep disorder may be extensive. Most sleep disorders are classified into disorders of insomnia, SRBDs, nocturnal movement or behavioral disorders, and disorders of hypersomnolence.

The clinical approach to patients presenting with a chief complaint of a sleep disorder begins with a comprehensive sleep history. Information, including the onset of symptoms, duration of symptoms, exacerbating and relieving factors, and whether complaints are from patients themselves or from a bed partner, is elicited. If a concern is a nocturnal behavior, such as snoring, irregular breathing patterns, excessive movement, or unusual behaviors, the descriptive detail provided by the patient, bed partner, or even audiovisual recordings is helpful. Additional details include a patient's daily schedule, usual bedtime, time to fall asleep, nocturnal awakenings, time to return to sleep, awakening time, estimated sleep time, and sense of sleep quality. Environmental factors, including light, noise, temperature, comfort of the bed, use of electronic devices, and pets, are all potential exacerbating factors. Morning symptoms, such as dry mouth, headache, jaw discomfort, and level of alertness, may assist with better defining a sleep problem. The daytime schedule, including naps, meal times, caffeine and alcohol use, and level of alertness, are also valuable. Review of past medical illnesses, medications, and social and family history and a review of systems should be routinely performed. For disorders suggestive of SRBDs, a detailed examination that, at a minimum, includes the upper airway, pulmonary, cardiovascular, and neurologic systems is recommended.

The authors have nothing to disclose.
Somnos Sleep Disorders Center, 1101 South 70th Street, Suite 102, Lincoln, NE 68510, USA
* Corresponding author.
E-mail address: jtrapp@somnos.com

Once an initial evaluation is complete, a differential diagnosis is created. The *International Classification of Sleep Disorders, Second Edition*, provides a comprehensive list of sleep diagnoses and presenting symptoms and is recommended for reference. Many sleep disorders may be easily identified and treated without additional testing. Use of sleep diaries, sleep questionnaires, overnight oximetry, laboratory testing, and imaging studies may be helpful in the appropriate clinical setting. Other disorders, such as SRBDs, require a more direct assessment of a patient's sleep. This is best performed through the PSG.

The PSG is the most commonly used test in the diagnosis of SRBDs. The PSG is considered the gold standard for the diagnosis of SRBDs and is useful in the evaluation and diagnosis of other sleep disorders. The PSG is indicated in the following diagnostic evaluations[1]:

- Diagnosis of SRBDs
- Positive airway pressure (PAP) and oral appliance therapy (OAT) titration in SRBDs
- Assessment of non-PAP treatment response of SRBDs
- Narcolepsy (PSG with multiple sleep latency test)
- Parasomnias that are complex or violent
- Seizure disorders (in circumstances where the clinical assessment or diagnostic electroencephalogram [EEG] is inconclusive)
- Periodic limb movement disorder.

PSG is not routinely recommended for disorders of insomnia, restless legs syndrome, circadian rhythm disorders, or depression.

PSG REFERRAL

Ordering a PSG requires referral to a designated sleep center. Referral may be directed first to a sleep specialist to provide further evaluation, diagnostic testing, education, and implementation of treatment. If PSG is indicated, the sleep specialist then may interpret the PSG with full knowledge of the patient who is evaluated and review the results with the patient before making treatment decisions. The sleep specialist may then provide longitudinal follow-up of the patient's condition, including response and adherence to therapy.

Referral may also be made directly to the sleep center for PSG testing by a primary health care provider or dental professional. The PSG is reviewed in context of the history and physical findings reported by the referring provider. An interpretation of the PSG with treatment suggestions is made available. If a treatment regimen or follow-up is beyond the scope of practice for the referring provider, sleep specialist consultation or other specialty consultation is recommended.

Selecting a Sleep Laboratory

Laboratories that perform sleep studies are commonly referred to as sleep centers to indicate facilities that are capable of evaluating and treating a full range of sleep disorders. Sleep centers may be accredited or unaccredited. The American Academy of Sleep Medicine (AASM) is the largest accrediting organization for sleep centers at present. According to the AASM, there are currently more than 2200 sleep centers in the United States that are AASM accredited.[2]

AASM accreditation requires adherence to specific standards in the areas of

- Personnel
- Policies and procedures

- Facility and equipment
- Patient evaluation and care
- Emergency procedures
- Data acquisition, scoring, and reporting
- Quality assurance.

An AASM-accredited sleep center must have a certified sleep specialist as medical director and must employ at least one registered sleep technologist. Accredited centers may be affiliated with a hospital or be independent, freestanding facilities. The AASM also offers accreditation for facilities that perform out-of-center sleep testing (ie, in-home testing) and for centers that offer durable medical equipment services (eg, continuous PAP [CPAP] equipment).[3]

Role of the Sleep Technologist

The PSG is a time-intensive and technically demanding diagnostic test. These recordings are performed by PSG technologists, commonly referred to as sleep technologists. Working under the supervision of a licensed physician, a sleep technologist assists in the clinical assessment of patients by means of screening questionnaires, physiologic monitoring, and testing (PSG); treatment of sleep disorders using various therapeutic tools, including PAP devices; and providing education and instruction to patients in their care.

Since 1979, the Board of Registered Polysomnographic Technologists has been the primary credentialing program for sleep technologists employed in the United States and many other countries around the world. The registered polysomnographic technologist (RPSGT) credential is held by more than 16,000 individuals and is widely recognized in the field of sleep technology. The RPSGT designation is obtained through completion of a formal training program, hands-on training experience in a sleep center, and successful completion of the certification examination.

In 2007 the National Board for Respiratory Care developed a sleep disorders specialty credential (registered respiratory therapist-sleep disorder specialist [RRT-SDS]), and in November of 2011, the AASM began offering an registered sleep technologists (RST) credentialing examination.

Role of the Sleep Specialist

Sleep specialists receive specialized education in the diagnosis and management of sleep disorders. Accreditation previously was obtained through the American Board of Sleep Medicine. In 2007, member boards of the American Board of Medical Specialties began administration of a subspecialty certification examination for sleep medicine. Member boards include the American Board of Anesthesiology, American Board of Family Medicine, American Board of Internal Medicine, American Board of Pediatrics, American Board of Psychiatry and Neurology, and the American Board of Otolaryngology. Currently, subspecialty certification may only be obtained through successful completion of a 12-month formal sleep medicine training program and acceptable performance on the sleep medicine certification examination. This is a time-limited certification and requires continuing medical education and periodic renewal every 10 years with a recertification examination.

Additional training provides sleep specialists with the knowledge base necessary for comprehensive PSG analysis and interpretation. The field of sleep disorders crosses many different specialties and thus makes necessary a diverse spectrum of treatment options.

THE POLYSOMNOGRAM

A PSG is the continuous recording of multiple physiologic variables over a sleep period that provides quantitative and qualitative measures of sleep. In the early days of sleep technology, the PSG recording was made on paper using a multichannel polygraph machine. PSGs are now routinely recorded using digital amplifiers and stored electronically (**Fig. 1**).

In-Center Polysomnogram

In-center PSGs are typically recorded during an overnight stay at the sleep center and monitored by a sleep technologist stationed in a nearby control room. When a patient sleeps during the day due to shift work, a PSG may be performed during the patient's usual bedtime hours.

Prestudy procedures include review of the order and indications for PSG; review of recent history and examination as provided by the referring health care provider; review of recent sleep diary, sleep questionnaires, medications, caffeine or alcohol consumption; and any change in a patient's overall health and schedule of activities in the days leading up to the PSG. Once the patient is ready, the hookup for PSG is initiated, during which various sensors are applied.

Electroencephalogram, Electro-oculogram, and Electromyography

EEG is the recording of surface electrical activity of the brain. Proper locations for EEG leads are determined by measuring a patient's head using the International 10–20 System of Electrode Placement. A standard PSG may use 4 to 6 scalp electrodes, plus references, for recording brain activity. EEG recording assists with determining sleep staging and wakefulness. More detailed EEG recording is obtained when there is clinical concern for seizure disorder.

Electro-oculography (EOG) is a recording of eye movements during sleep and wakefulness. Eye movements are recorded as deflections in the EOG leads. EOG allows

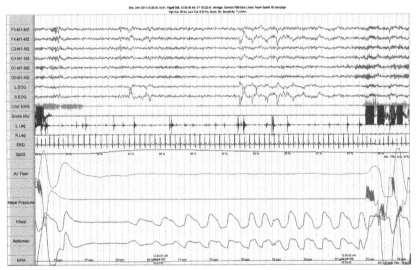

Fig. 1. A 60-second sample of an in-center attended PSG showing a mixed apnea during stage R (REM) sleep, concluding with an arousal.

identification of phasic bursts in rapid eye movements (REMs) that characterize this stage of sleep. Slow lateral eye movements may be the first manifestation of drowsiness helping to better identify sleep onset.

Leads are also placed for the recording of electromyography (EMG) activity in the chin or submental region. Submental EMG is helpful in the assessment of snoring, bruxism, and sleep stage scoring. High chin EMG tone is generally observed with wakefulness, movement, snoring, and bruxism. Typically the chin EMG tone is lowest during REM sleep.

Bilateral leg EMG recordings are useful in the diagnosis of periodic limb movements of sleep (PLMS). Additional limb EMG recordings are obtained in special circumstances.

Electrocardiogram

A single channel of electrocardiographic (ECG) activity is generally recorded using the lead II placement (right arm to left hip) giving the technologist and sleep specialist the ability to identify common cardiac arrhythmias.

Respiratory variables

Airflow variables are measured with a thermal mouth/nose sensor and nasal pressure canula. Thoracic and abdominal belts are worn by patients to record respiratory effort. An oximetry probe is used to continuously measure oxygen saturation and may be affixed to a finger or ear lobe. In addition to these recording variables, additional devices can be used to monitor end-tidal CO_2 and/or esophageal pressure. Recording of airflow, respiratory effort, and oximetry is necessary in the diagnosis of SRBDs.

Audio and video monitoring

Breath sounds, body position, and unusual behaviors or movements occurring during sleep can be recorded by means of video and audio monitoring equipment in the patient bedroom or via first-hand observation and documentation by a sleep technologist.

Body position is particularly helpful in assessment of SRBDs. Frequently, these disorders are more severe while in supine sleep, likely related to jaw and tongue position and posterior displacement, resulting in more severe obstruction. In some cases, position retraining alone to avoid the supine position may be helpful in the treatment of an SRBD.

Pretest calibration

On completion of the sensor application, electrode impedances are checked to confirm proper site preparation and adequate contact with the skin before the start of the PSG recording. A sleep technologist performs a mechanical calibration of the recording equipment and then a physiologic calibration by giving a patient various commands to confirm the correct function of certain sensors. An example is the calibration of the EOG channels, which may include having a patient open and close the eyes and look left and right and up and down.

A typical recording montage for an attended, clinical PSG performed in a sleep center is shown in **Table 1**.

Split-Night PSG

A clinical PSG that combines a diagnostic study with a titration study in a single night is often called a split-night study. This type of study is performed when the first 2 or 3 hours of the PSG yields an elevated apnea hypopnea index (AHI) sufficient to begin therapy. The remainder of the sleep time is then used to titrate therapy in the form of PAP or oral appliance device. A recent clinical study has confirmed that the AHI

Table 1		
PSG recording montage		
Channel No.	**Category**	**Derivation or Device**
1	Left frontal lobe EEG	F3–M2
2	Right frontal lobe EEG	F4–M1
3	Left central lobe EEG	C3–M2
4	Right central lobe EEG	C4–M1
5	Left occipital lobe EEG	O1–M2
6	Right occipital lobe EEG	O2–M1
7	Left EOG	LOC–M2
8	Right EOG	ROC–M1
9	Submental EMG	EMG leads on the chin/jaw
10	Left leg EMG	EMG leads on the left anterior tibialis
11	Right leg EMG	EMG leads on the right anterior tibialis
12	ECG	Lead II ECG
13	Oral/nasal airflow	Oral/nasal thermocouple
14	Nasal pressure	Nasal pressure transducer
15	Thoracic effort	Inductance plethysmography belt
16	Abdominal effort	Inductance plethysmography belt
17	Oxygen saturation	Pulse oximetry probe
18	Heart rate (bpm)	Pulse oximetry probe

Abbreviations: bpm, beats per minute; LOC, left outer canthus; ROC, right outer canthus.

obtained in the first few hours of sleep in patients suspected of having an SRBD is an accurate representation of the AHI from a full night PSG.[4] Many sleep centers follow the current Centers for Medicare & Medicaid Services (CMS) guideline of an estimated AHI greater than or equal to 15 or a minimum of 30 scored apnea hypopnea events within 2 hours to initiate a split-night study.[5] For most patients, PAP titration is performed unless prior fitting for an oral appliance device has been done. Split-night studies provide convenience for patients and may reduce the overall cost of care for treatment of SRBDs.

Out-of-Center PSG

An out-of-center PSG is an unattended study performed to confirm the diagnosis of SRBDs in medically stable patients with a high pretest probability of moderate to severe SRBDs. Some unattended PSG recording systems are able to obtain data similar to an attended, in-center PSG. But many out-of-center studies, for simplicity, limit data collection to respiratory-related signals, including nasal pressure, respiratory effort, pulse rate, and oxygen saturation.

Patients undergoing out-of-center PSG are given advance instruction on the self-application of the study sensors and are also responsible for starting and stopping the study on the recording device. The recording device is then returned to the sleep center for data analysis and interpretation.

The PSG Report

An initial method for assessing the sleep cycle on a single night study is through review of the sleep hypnogram. This provides a graphic representation of the sleep stages and sleep cycles as well as a general overview of the scored sleep-related events. These may include SRBD events, arousals, and limb movements. This overview assists clinicians in obtaining an overall assessment of the PSG. **Fig. 2** shows a sample PSG report, including a sleep hypnogram.

Scoring rules for PSGs are based on published guidelines implemented by the AASM.[6] Detailed PSG data are generally tabulated in a report produced by a scoring sleep technologist and include quantitative and qualitative measures, including sleep staging, respiratory events, limb movements, ECG events, arousals, breath sounds, and comments. Definitions for common sleep parameters are given in **Table 2**.[7]

Sleep Staging

EEG, EOG, and chin EMG are required to accurately score sleep stages. Sleep stage scoring is performed in 30-second epochs. An epoch is assigned a sleep stage based on the predominant sleep stage pattern present on that epoch. Sleep stages are divided into 5 categories:

- W (wake)
- N1 (non-REM stage 1)
- N2 (non-REM stage 2)
- N3 (non-REM stage 3)
- R (REM stage sleep).

For normal, young adult patients, sleep stages progress in a predictable manner starting with a few minutes of N1 sleep on sleep onset followed sequentially by N2, N3, and R sleep. This cycle lasts approximately 90 minutes and may repeat 4 to 6 times during the night. Periods of N3 sleep decrease as the night progresses, whereas stage R sleep periods lengthen with each successive sleep cycle. Expected proportions of the 4 sleep stages are as follows[8]:

N1—5% to 10% of total sleep time (TST)
N2—50% to 60% of TST
N3—10% to 20% of TST
R—20% to 25% of TST.

Sleep latencies and sleep efficiency may vary considerably by age; however, a sleep-onset latency of less than 30 minutes is generally considered normal and the first cycle of REM sleep usually occurs between 60 and 120 minutes after sleep onset. Sleep efficiency of 85% or greater is expected in most normal sleepers but may be reduced in older adults.[9]

Respiratory Events

The respiratory portion of the PSG identifies and quantifies respiratory events. Recognized respiratory events commonly include apneas, hypopneas, and respiratory effort–related arousals (RERAs). An apnea is defined as the complete cessation of airflow for a minimum of 10 seconds regardless of whether or not there is an associated oxygen desaturation.[10] Apneas are classified as obstructive if there is respiratory effort identified and central if no respiratory effort is identified.[1] Mixed apneas are identified if there is initial absence of airflow followed by initiation of respiratory effort before initiation of actual airflow.[6]

A hypopnea is defined as an event with a 30% or greater decrease in the nasal pressure signal lasting at least 10 seconds accompanied by a minimum 4% decrease in the blood oxygen level.[11]

ABC Sleep Center   **Phone: XXX-XXX-XXXX**

Patient Name: Smith, Mary A.   DOB: XX/XX/XXXX   Date of Study: XX/XX/XXXX

Reason for Study: Ms. Smith is a 60-year-old female with history of an abnormal overnight oximetry study. She describes snoring, nocturnal gasping or choking for air, and mild daytime hypersomnolence. Medical history is remarkable for hypertension.

General Summary

Date of Study:	XX/XX/XXXX	**Epoch Length:**	30 Seconds
Lights Out:	9:48:35 PM	**Lights On:**	5:15:35 AM
Recording Time (TRT):	459.5 min. (7.7 hrs.)	**Time Out of Bed:**	0.0 min.
Time in Bed (TIB):	447.0 min.	**Awake Time in Bed:**	87.5 min.
Total Sleep Time (TST):	359.5 min. (6.0 hrs.)	**Sleep Efficiency:**	80 %

Sleep Stage Summary

Sleep Stages	Time (min)	% TST	% TIB
N1	18.5 min.	5 %	4%
N2	191.0 min.	53 %	43%
N3	72.0 min.	20 %	16%
REM	78.0 min.	22 %	17%
Wake	87.5 min.		20%
Totals	7.66Hrs.	6.0 Hrs.	7.5 Hrs.

Latency from Lights Out

Latency to N1	6.0 min.
Latency to REM	89.0 min

Respiratory Events

NREM	Central Apnea	Obstructive Apnea	Mixed Apnea	Hypopnea	RERA
Occurrences	0	3	0	31	3
Max. Duration (sec.)	0.0	35.8	0.0	33.6	6
Mean Duration (sec.)	0.0	26.2	0.0	23.1	6
NREM Index	0	0.6	0.0	6.6	0.6

REM	Central Apnea	Obstructive Apnea	Mixed Apnea	Hypopnea	RERA
Occurrences	1	0	0	52	0
Max. Duration (sec.)	12.5	0.0	0.0	75.1	0
Mean Duration (sec.)	12.5	0.0	0.0	31.3	0
REM Index	1	0.0	0.0	40.0	0.0

Total Sleep Time	Central Apnea	Obstructive Apnea	Mixed Apnea	Hypopnea	RERA
Occurrences	1	3	0	83	3
Max. Duration (sec.)	12.5	35.8	0.0	75.1	6
Mean Duration (sec.)	12.5	26.2	0.0	28.3	6
Total Index	0	0.5	0.0	13.9	0.4

	NREM	REM	Total
AHI	7	41	15
RDI	8	41	15

AHI by Position

Position (min.)	TIB (min.)	REM (min.)	NREM (min.)	Apnea/ Hypopnea C / O / M / H	AHI	Mean SpO2 % Sleep	Snore Index
Supine	125.4	18.0	79.5	0 / 2 / 0 / 34	22	91 %	1
Left	196.8	46.0	130.5	1 / 1 / 0 / 38	14	91 %	1
Prone	0.0	0.0	0.0	0 / 0 / 0 / 0	0	0 %	0

Fig. 2. A PSG report with hypnogram.

Right	124.8	14.0	71.5	0 / 0 / 0 / 11	8	92 %	1
Upright	0.0	0.0	0.0	0 / 0 / 0 / 0	0	0 %	0
Non-supine	321.6	60.0	202.0	1/1/0/49	11.7	91%	1

Oximetry Summary

	Total	REM	NREM	Awake
<50%	0.0 min.	0.0 min.	0.0 min.	0.0 min.
51 – 60%	0.0 min.	0.0 min.	0.0 min.	0.0 min.
61 – 70%	0.0 min.	0.0 min.	0.0 min.	0.0 min.
71 – 80%	0.4 min.	0.4 min.	0.0 min.	0.0 min.
81 – 90%	113.8 min.	26.5 min.	78.8 min.	8.5 min.
91 - 100%	325.3 min.	51.1 min.	201.5 min.	72.7 min.
Average	91	91	91	92
Minimum SpO2	77	77	87	82
Desaturation Event Index	0.0	0.0	0.0	0.0
# Desat. Events below 89%	0	0	0	0
Time(%) with Saturation below 89%	3.9	2.5	0.7	0.6
Time(min.) with Saturation below 89%	17.1	11.2	3.0	2.8

Arousal

	REM	NREM	Total
Arousals with Respiratory Events:	9	4	13
Arousals with Limb Movement Events:	0	18	18
Arousals with Snoring Events:	2	3	5
Non-Specific Arousals:	8	32	42
Total Arousals:	20	58	78
Arousal Index:	15	12	13

Snoring Data

	REM	NREM	Total
Total Snoring Time (min):	41.5	87.3	128.8

Cardiac Events

	NREM	REM	WAKE
Mean Heart Rate (bpm):	58	59	62
Low Heart Rate (bpm):	50	51	52
High Heart Rate (bpm):	109	75	107

PLMS

	In Episodes	Not In Episodes	Total
Total Limb Movements	162	15	178
Limb Movement Index	27.0	2.0	29.5
Limb Movements with Arousal Index	2.3	0.7	3.0

Fig. 2. (*continued*)

RERA events are usually not associated with oxygen desaturation but in some individuals may manifest similar symptoms of fatigue or sleepiness as patients with obstructive sleep apnea.[11] A RERA is defined as a period of 10 seconds or more of increasing effort or flattening of the nasal pressure signal leading to an arousal from sleep. An event that meets criteria for an apnea or hypopnea cannot be a RERA. RERA events are best detected with an esophageal manometer, but nasal pressure and respiratory inductance plethysmography belts may also be used.[6]

AHI and RDI

The AHI is the average number of apneas and hypopneas per hour of sleep and is used to diagnose and assist in defining the severity of an SRBD.

Hypnogram

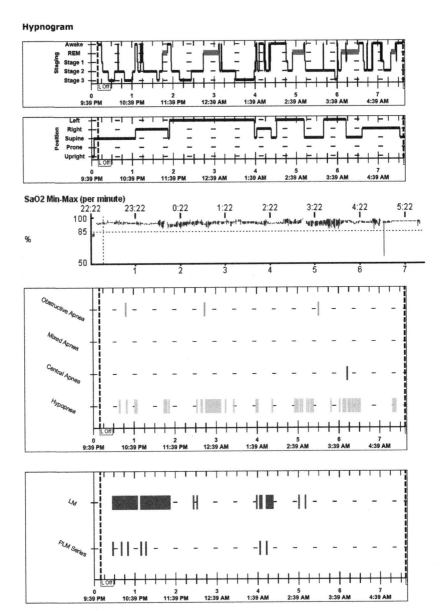

Fig. 2. (continued)

Table 2 Sleep parameter definitions	
Term	**Definition**
Epoch	30-Second period of recording
TRT	Total recording time or time in bed from lights out to lights on
TST	Total sleep time during the recording
Sleep Efficiency	TST as a percentage of TRT
SOL	Sleep onset latency or time from lights out until sleep onset
REM Latency	Time from sleep onset to the first epoch of stage R sleep

Mild sleep apnea $5 \leq AHI \leq 15$
Moderate sleep apnea $15 < AHI \leq 30$
Severe sleep apnea $AHI > 30$.

Although this classification is commonly used, no general consensus of severity classification has been established. Many other parameters are believed to contribute to the severity of SRBDs, including oxygen desaturations, cardiac dysrhythmias, comorbid medical conditions, and clinical symptoms of daytime sleepiness and cognitive function.

A CMS-approved definition of SRBD is defined as[5]

- AHI or RDI ≥ 15 events per hour or
- AHI or RDI ≥ 5 and ≤ 14 events per hour with documented symptoms of excessive daytime sleepiness, impaired cognition, mood disorders or insomnia, or documented hypertension, ischemic heart disease, or history of stroke.

The respiratory disturbance index (RDI) is the average number of apneas, hypopopneas, and RERAs per hour of sleep. Upper airway resistance syndrome has been traditionally defined as AHI less than 5 and RERAs as the predominant respiratory finding on PSG.[11]

Electrocardiogram

Cardiac monitoring of the heart rhythm during the PSG is with a single lead ECG recording, usually lead II. The most significant rhythm disturbances that occur during the PSG are commonly related to SRBDs. During cycles of SRBDs, episodes of hypoxemia followed by reoxygenation, cyclic hypercapnea and hypocapnea, and fluctuations in intrathoracic pressure adversely effect cardiovascular function.[12] In some patients, an apnea may be associated with bradycardia (slowing of the heart rhythm) followed by tachycardia (acceleration of the heart rhythm) once breathing is reinitiated. This pattern manifests as a cyclical bradycardia-tachycardia arrhythmia through the study.[12] Bradycardia may be especially severe and in some cases this may result in sinus arrest,[13–15] which is a prolonged pause of the normal heart rhythm. These rhythms may occur in patients with normal heart function.[14] In some patients, prolonged heart rhythm pauses, resulting in hypoperfusion may have a pronounced effect on the ischemic heart and may result in ventricular arrhythmias.[14,16] Treatment of the SRBDs with a device, such as CPAP, results in resolution of most of these cardiac events.[14,16]

Atrial fibrillation is associated with SRBDs.[14,17] Correction of SRBDs may result in a marked improvement in the successful treatment of this arrhythmia.[18] Patients with atrial fibrillation and other serious arrhythmias should be screened for SRBDs.

Limb Movements

PLMS are characterized by episodes of repetitive, stereotyped limb movements and are a common finding on the PSG.[19–21] Typical movements may be rhythmic extension of the first toe or dorsiflexion of the ankle. These manifest on a PSG as brief repetitive muscle movements on the leg EMG. Scoring criteria for PLMS are defined by the AASM scoring manual.[6,21] PLMS may occur in several different sleep disorders, including SRBDs, but commonly occur in patients with a diagnosis of restless legs syndrome.[22] PLMS, however, are frequently identified in asymptomatic patients and seem to increase in frequency with age.[23] The mean number of PLMS per hour is defined as the PLMS index. When PLMS are associated with arousal, a PLM with arousal index may also be calculated. A PLM index, with or without arousal, greater than 15 events per hour, is considered abnormal in adults.[24] When PLMS are associated with related sleep complaints, this may be called a periodic limb movement disorder. Several studies, however, question the significance of PLMS and their impact on sleep complaints.[25–27] Evaluation and treatment decisions are frequently based on the perceived impact on sleep and the association with restless legs syndrome.

SUMMARY

The evaluation of patients presenting with sleep disorders is complex, requiring an investigative approach that synthesizes information obtained through a detailed history, focused physical examination, and appropriate confirmatory testing. The PSG is the only clinical tool that measures multiple physiologic variables to qualitatively and quantitatively evaluate sleep. A proper understanding of the role of PSG, its measurements, and interpretation allows for a proper diagnosis so as to provide an optimal range of treatments for individual patients.

REFERENCES

1. Kushida C, Littner M, Morgenthaler T, et al. Practice parameters for the indications for polysomnography and related procedures: an update for 2005. Sleep 2005;28(4):499–521.
2. American Academy of Sleep Medicine Web site. Available at: http://www.aasmnet.org/members/resources/pdf/innovationproposal.pdf. 2011. p. 4. Accessed November 8, 2011.
3. American Academy of Sleep Medicine Web site. Available at: http://www.aasmnet.org/Resources/PDF/AASMcenteraccredstandards.pdf. 2011. Accessed November 8, 2011.
4. Khawaja I, Olson E, van der Walt C, et al. Diagnostic accuracy of split-night polysomnograms. J Clin Sleep Med 2010;6(4):357–62.
5. Noridian Administrative Services Web site. Available at: https://www.noridianmedicare/com/dme/coverage/docs/lcds/current_lcds/positive_airway_pressure_pap_devices_for_the_treatment_of_obstructive_sleep_apnea.htm%3f. 2011. Accessed November 8, 2011.
6. The AASM manual for the scoring of sleep and associated events. Westchester (IL): American Academy of Sleep Medicine; 2007.
7. Mattice C. Sleep report parameters and calculations. Respir Care Clin N Am 2006;12:13.
8. Bixler EO, Vela-Bueno A. Normal sleep: patterns and mechanisms. Semin Neurol 1987;7(3):228.

9. Hirshkowitz M, Moore CA, Hamilton CR III, et al. Polysomnography of adults and elderly: sleep architecture, respiration, and leg movement. J Clin Neurophysiol 1992;9(1):59.
10. Butkov N. Atlas of clinical polysomnography, vol. II. Ashland (OR): Synapse Media; 1996. p. 184–9.
11. Guilleminault C, Stoohs R, Clerk A, et al. A cause of excessive daytime sleepiness: the upper airway resistance syndrome. Chest 1993;104:184–9.
12. Somers V, Javaheri S. Cardiovascular effects of sleep-related breathing disorders. 4th edition. St Louis (MO): Principles and practice of sleep medicine; 2005. p. 1180–91.
13. Guilleminault C, Connolly S, Winkle R, et al. Cyclical variation of the heart rate in sleep apnea syndrome: mechanisms, and usefulness of 24 h electrocardiography as a screening technique. Lancet 1984;1:126–31.
14. Guilleminault C, Connolly S, Winkle R, et al. Cardiac arrhythmia and conduction disturbances during sleep in 400 patients with sleep apnea syndrome. Am J Cardiol 1983;52:490–4.
15. Zwillich C, Devlin T, White D, et al. Bradycardia during sleep apnea: characteristics and mechanism. J Clin Invest 1983;69:1286–92.
16. Peled N, Abinnader E, Pillar G, et al. Nocturnal ischemia events in patients with obstructive sleep apnea syndrome and ischemic heart disease: effects of continuous positive airway pressure treatment. J Am Coll Cardiol 1999;34:1744–9.
17. Gami A, Pressman G, Caples S, et al. Association of atrial fibrillation and obstructive sleep apnea. Circulation 2004;110:364–7.
18. Kanagala R, Murali N, Friedman P, et al. Obstructive sleep apnea and the recurrence of atrial fibrillation. Circulation 2003;107:2589–94.
19. Coleman R. Periodic movements in sleep (nocturnal myoclonus) and restless legs syndrome. In: Guilleminault C, editor. Sleep and waking disorders: indications and techniques. Menlo Park (CA): Addison-wesley; 1982. p. 265–95.
20. American Sleep Disorders Association. Sleep disorders. EEG arousals: scoring rules and examples: a preliminary report from the sleep disorders atlas task force of the American Sleep Disorders Association. Sleep 1992;15:173–84.
21. Zucconi M, Ferri R, Allen R, et al. The official world association of sleep medicine (WASM) standards for recording and scoring periodic leg movements in sleep (PLMS) and wakefulness (PLMW) developed in collaboration with a task force from the international restless legs syndrome study group (IRLSSG). Sleep 2006;7:175–83.
22. Lugaresi E, Cirignotta F, Coccagna G, et al. Nocturnal myoclonus and restless legs syndrome. Adv Neurol 1986;43:295–307.
23. Ancoli-Israël S, Kripke D, Mason W, et al. Sleep apnea and periodic movements in sleep in an aging population. J Gerontol 1985;40:419–25.
24. The international classification of sleep disorders. 2nd edition. Westchester (IL): American Academy of Sleep Medicine; 2005.
25. Montplaiser J, Michaud M, Denesle R, et al. Periodic leg movements are not more prevalent in insomnia or hypersomnia but are specifically associated with sleep disorders involving a dopaminergic impairment. Sleep 2000;1:163–7.
26. Coleman R, Pollak C, Weitzman E. Periodic movements in sleep (nocturnal myoclonus): relation to sleep disorders. Ann Neurol 1980;8:416–21.
27. Karadeniz D, Ondze B, Besset A, et al. Are periodic leg movements during sleep (PLMS) responsible for sleep disruption in insomnia patients? Eur J Neurol 2000; 7:331–6.

Medical Disorders Impacted by Obstructive Sleep Apnea

Sabin R. Bista, MBBS*, Teri J. Barkoukis, MD

KEYWORDS

- Obstructive sleep apnea • Continuous positive airway pressure
- OSA medical complications

Normal sleeping individuals experience a lower metabolic rate and relative cardiovascular quiescent state with lower heart rate and blood pressure that naturally occurs during sleep compared with the waking state. In patients with obstructive sleep apnea (OSA), this quiescent state becomes disrupted. Research has shown a higher risk for several medical disorders, most ominous being a myocardial infarction or stroke. This article serves as an overview to the cardiovascular, cerebrovascular, metabolic, and gastroesophageal effects of OSA.

OVERVIEW OF PATHOPHYSIOLOGY

Complete pathophysiology and background of disease mechanisms is beyond the scope of this article; however, a brief introduction may be helpful before introducing each medical complication of sleep apnea. Please see **Fig. 1** for a graphical representation[1] of the following succinct explanation.

Most patients with sleep apnea trigger hypoxemic events during the apnea with reoxygenation on recovery from the apnea event, causing oxidative stress. Intermittent hypoxia can potentially lead to reactive oxygen species that can damage biomolecules and alter cellular functions that can contribute to inflammation and endothelial dysfunction.[2] The longer the period of apnea, the more likely transient hypercapnia can also result. It has also been well described that sleep apnea increases sympathetic activation[3] leading to vasoconstriction, a strong factor in cardiovascular consequences of sleep apnea. Inflammation including elevations of C-reactive protein (CRP),[4,5] adhesion molecules, and other cytokines and inflammatory mediators has been shown to be overly active in patients with sleep apnea.[1,6] Although platelet dysfunction and factors of coagulation, such as fibrinogen, are increased in patients

The authors have nothing to disclose.
Division of Pulmonary, Critical Care, Sleep and Allergy, University of Nebraska Medical Center, Box 985300, Nebraska Medical Center, Omaha, NE 68198-5300, USA
* Corresponding author.
E-mail address: sbista@unmc.edu

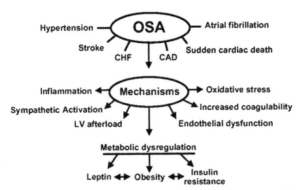

Fig. 1. Association between OSA and cardiovascular disease; partial list of the disease mechanisms associated with OSA considered as possible links to several cardiovascular diseases and metabolic dysregulation. CAD, coronary artery disease; CHF, congestive heart failure; LV, left ventricular. (*Reprinted from* Lopez-Jimenez F, Sert Kuniyoshi FH, Gami A, et al. Obstructive sleep apnea: implications for cardiac and vascular disease. Chest 2008; 133:793–804; with permission.)

with sleep apnea,[7] the clear connection to sleep apnea as a direct cause is not certain and may be linked to other comorbid conditions.

Each obstructive apnea is accompanied by waves of effort against a closed airway that, in turn, causes negative intrathoracic pressure changes. Transmural pressure increases across the heart and great vessels with a ripple effect of increased afterload, atrial size, diastolic dysfunction, and increased cardiac wall stress.[6,8,9]

Leptin, a protein involved in appetite suppression, has been shown to be elevated in patients with OSA at levels higher than in subjects with a comparable body mass index (BMI).[10] Other important metabolic dysregulation has a connection between relative insulin resistance and patients with sleep apnea. This glucose intolerance associated with OSA appears to be independent of BMI.[11–13]

CARDIOVASCULAR
Systemic Hypertension

Important information to understand the link between systemic hypertension and patients with sleep apnea has been evident in several studies. The Wisconsin Sleep Cohort Study showed a dose-response relationship between OSA and blood pressure elevations independent of age, sex, BMI, and other factors.[14] It is interesting to note that the Sleep Heart Health Study did not show a statistical difference once BMI was factored out, with the implication that the development of hypertension was more related to obesity itself rather than purely OSA.[15] There were enough differences in study design, for example, using a different score for apnea-hypopnea index (AHI), so as not to discount a link with systemic hypertension; however, there are likely other associated factors.[16] Nonetheless, the seventh Joint National Committee on Prevention, Detection, Evaluation, and Treatment of High Blood Pressure stated the importance of OSA as a risk factor for systemic hypertension.[17]

Intermittent nocturnal hypoxia not only sets off oxidative stress and other factors introduced earlier, but also activates the renin-angiotensin system. This then increases endothelin-I, an amino acid peptide produced by vascular endothelial cells and an important vasoconstrictor in the pathway leading to systemic hypertension.[18] Angiotensin II, a bioactive product of the renin-angiotensin system, is a potent arteriole vasoconstrictor and triggers release of aldosterone that can lead to fluid accumulation and further airway resistance.[18–20]

Continuous positive airway pressure (CPAP) has been shown to improve blood pressure control in hypertensive patients. A recent small study revealed that CPAP therapy in a small group of hypertensive subjects reduced sympathetic activity during the daytime and reduced vascular resistance.[21] Another larger prospective controlled study showed data to suggest that OSA is associated with increased arterial stiffness that was independent of age, gender, BMI, antihypertensive medications, and hypertension and that CPAP therapy significantly reduced arterial stiffness.[22] If a patient with elevated blood pressure cannot tolerate CPAP, oral appliances have also recently been shown to improve hypertension in small studies.[23,24]

Myocardial Ischemia and Infarction

There is evidence of a greater prevalence of OSA in patients with coronary artery disease than those who do not have coronary artery disease. As mentioned earlier, intermittent hypoxia as a result of sleep apnea in the face of a reduction of stroke volume in combination with cardiac transmural pressure elevation in susceptible patients with coronary artery disease can lead to increased risk of myocardial infarction and sudden death. Other factors include blood pressure surges with the sympathetic activation and intrathoracic pressure swings, systemic inflammation, and endothelial dysfunction.[5,6,25] **Table 1** lists the process from pathophysiology to subsequent disease.

When patients with OSA were compared with control subjects, there were more episodes of cardiac arrhythmias and nocturnal ST-segment depression.[26] Peker and colleagues[27] reported, on a study of 182 men with and without OSA over 7 years, an increased risk of developing cardiovascular disease that was independent of age, BMI, blood pressure, and smoking. A larger study of participants followed over a 10-year period showed a significant increase in both fatal and nonfatal cardiovascular events in patients with severe OSA who were on no therapy compared with healthy controls.[28] CPAP therapy for patients with OSA with ischemic heart disease has been shown to lessen the severity of ST-segment depression.[29] Despite growing evidence of nocturnal cardiac ischemia in patients with OSA, a small study of patients with coronary artery disease with moderate or severe OSA did not show detectable myocardial injury by cardiac troponin T assay.[30] Another study also mentioned that cardiac troponin assay remained unchanged; however, CRP served as a useful cardiac biomarker. CRP correlated with improved systolic and diastolic cardiac function and overall cardiovascular remodeling in patients with OSA on CPAP therapy.[31]

Table 1		
Mechanisms of myocardial ischemia and infarction in patients with sleep apnea		
Underlying Pathophysiology	**Signs and Symptoms**	**Disease Progression**
Profound intermittent hypoxia	Nocturnal angina (symptoms	Coronary artery disease
Sympathetic vasoconstriction	of chest discomfort)	Ventricular arrhythmias
Cellular level acidosis	Nocturnal ST depression on	Myocardial ischemia
Blood pressure elevation	electrocardiogram	Myocardial infarction
Endothelial dysfunction		Sudden cardiac death[a]
Systemic inflammation		
↑Cardiac transmural pressure		

[a] Sudden cardiac death timing is traditionally between the hours of 6 and 11 AM; however, in those with OSA, this shifts over to traditional sleeping periods, most pronounced between 12 midnight and 6 AM.[94]

Cardiac Arrhythmias

Some cardiac arrhythmias can occur during sleep in healthy individuals, including premature atrial contractions, premature ventricular contractions, and sinus pauses. Patients with OSA have been shown to have premature ventricular contractions, non-sustained ventricular tachycardia, bradyarrhythmias, sinus arrest, and second-degree atrioventricular block.[17,32,33] **Fig. 2** shows examples of various electrocardiographic (ECG) rhythms during sleep.[34]

Patients with OSA can have more arrhythmias that cause adverse health consequences than patients who do not have OSA. Atrial fibrillation (AF) has a higher

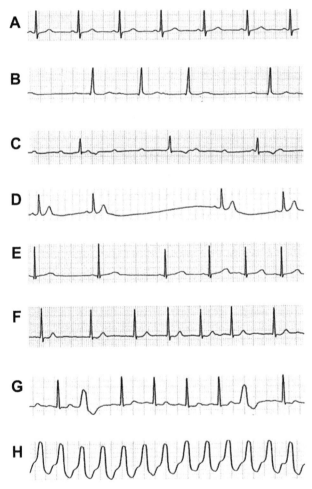

Fig. 2. Examples of various ECG rhythms that might be seen during sleep. (*A*) Normal sinus rhythm. (*B, C*) Atrioventricular conduction block: P wave is not followed by the QRS complex. (*D*) Sinus pause. (*E*) Atrial fibrillation: no P waves are visible. (*F*) Sinus arrhythmia. (*G*) Isolated extrasystoles. (*H*) Ventricular tachycardia. Note that the QRS complex is narrow in the supraventricular arrhythmias differentiating them from ventricular arrhythmias (in the absence of preexisting bundle branch block). (*Reprinted from* Hanak V, Konecny T, Somers VK. Cardiovascular pathophysiology of sleep apnea. In: Avidan AY, Barkoukis TJ, editors. Review of sleep medicine. Philadelphia: Elsevier-Saunders; 2011; with permission.)

incidence in patients with OSA. AF has a very high risk of recurrence after cardioversion unless the patient is on adequate OSA therapy.[35] Even after catheter ablation of AF, there is a 25% greater risk of recurring AF in patients with OSA than in those with no OSA.[36]

Pulmonary Hypertension

Pulmonary hypertension in subjects with OSA is likely attributable to hyper-reactivity to hypoxia, pulmonary arteriole remodeling, and impaired left ventricular diastolic function and enlarged left atria.[37] Although there are multiple pulmonary artery pressure elevations with OSA events, daytime sustained pulmonary hypertension as a result of sleep apnea has been less clearly linked. Patients with pulmonary hypertension and OSA tend to have more profound nocturnal hypoxemia, but may also have daytime hypoxemia as well, such as in obesity-hypoventilation syndrome or in patients who also have chronic obstructive pulmonary disease (COPD). Those patients with OSA with more predominant hypoxemia are at greater risk, as hypoxemia induces pulmonary artery pressure elevation. Despite controversy as to whether OSA is a primary cause of persistent pulmonary artery hypertension, CPAP has been shown to lower pulmonary artery pressure.[6,22,31,38]

STROKE

Stroke is a condition of acute injury to central nervous system tissue arising either from ischemia, which is more common, or hemorrhage. Transient ischemic attack (TIA) is a transient neurologic dysfunction secondary to focal ischemia but without infarction; however, it does increase the risk for stroke.[39] Stroke is a major health care problem in the United States, leading to many deaths, as well as functional impairment in survivors.[40] Both snoring and OSA have been linked to an increased incidence of stroke, and the risk for developing stroke increases with increased severity of sleep apnea at baseline.[41,42] The increased incidence is most likely secondary to interplay of various factors (see **Fig. 1**). OSA is known to contribute to increased risk for hypertension, cardiac arrhythmia, increased platelet adhesions, and dysfunction of vascular endothelium.[43,44] In fact, heavy snoring and OSA have been associated with increased risk for carotid atherosclerosis and arterial intima-media thickening.[45,46] Interestingly, stroke and TIA are risk factors for developing obstructive and central apneas as well. About half of patients who had an acute stroke have sleep apnea, and improvement is expected, more with central than obstructive apnea events, in only about half of patients in subsequent months.[47,48] Studies suggest that presence of moderate to severe OSA after stroke may lead to worse functional outcome and increase the risk for early death.[49,50] There are limited and conflicting data on outcome of positive airway pressure therapy for sleep apnea following stroke.[51,52]

DIABETES MELLITUS

There is a growing body of evidence from numerous human and animal studies that suggests an association between OSA and insulin resistance, glucose intolerance, and type 2 diabetes mellitus (DM2). Deficient insulin action lies at the heart of the problem in diabetes mellitus, which leads to hyperglycemia as a result of inadequate insulin secretion or diminished action on peripheral tissues, or both. The American Diabetes Association has established criteria to properly diagnose DM2 based on plasma glucose or hemoglobin A1C levels (**Box 1**).[53] An intermediate category is also recognized that puts an individual at risk for developing diabetes in the future. Prediabetes is the term often used to describe a clinical scenario where glucose levels

---

Box 1
American Diabetes Association criteria for diagnosing diabetes mellitus type 2

Hemoglobin A1C ≥6.5%

   OR

Fasting plasma glucose ≥126 mg

   OR

2-hour plasma glucose ≥200 mg/dL during oral glucose tolerance test

   OR

Random plasma glucose ≥200 mg/dL plus classic symptoms of hyperglycemia

---

are higher than normal but less than that used for diagnosing diabetes. Impaired fasting glucose and impaired glucose tolerance fall under this category (**Box 2**).[53,54]

Patients with concomitant OSA and DM2 are frequently encountered in clinical practice. Clinic-based cross-sectional studies have examined the relationship between polysomnography (PSG)-diagnosed OSA and glucose metabolism. Most studies have demonstrated impaired glucose tolerance, higher fasting glucose, and insulin resistance in patients with OSA compared with patients without OSA irrespective of weight, presence of visceral fat, and age.[55–57] In a clinic-based study of 595 men, OSA was diagnosed in 494 patients and 30.1% of these were found to have DM2, when diagnosed on the basis of 2-hour oral glucose tolerance test.[58] There are also population-based cross-sectional studies linking OSA to altered glucose metabolism and DM2. Some of these studies have used surrogate markers of OSA, such as snoring and witnessed apneas,[59–63] whereas others have diagnosed OSA by PSG.[12,64,65] A more robust association between OSA surrogate markers and DM2 has been shown by longitudinal studies. A 10-year follow-up study of 2668 Swedish men showed self-reported diabetes in 5.4% of habitual snorers at baseline compared with 2.4% without (P<.001). In addition, the occurrence of incident diabetes in obese snorers was 7 times more likely than nonobese snorers.[66] Likewise, in the US Nurses' Health Study involving 69,852 women where presence of DM2 was confirmed by composite clinical and laboratory criteria, there was a twofold increase in the risk of developing diabetes in habitual snorers at a 10-year follow-up even when adjusted for age, BMI, smoking history, number of sleep hours, history of hypertension, or family history of diabetes.[67] These studies suggest a causal relationship between OSA and diabetes mellitus, but are severely limited by the lack of PSG data. The available data on studies with OSA diagnosed by PSG is conflicting and limited by number of years of follow-up. Although one observational cohort study with a mean duration of

---

Box 2
Prediabetes criteria

Impaired fasting glucose: fasting plasma glucose 100–125 mg/dL

   OR

Impaired glucose tolerance: 2-hour plasma glucose 140–199 mg/dL oral glucose tolerance test

   OR

Hemoglobin A1C 5.7–6.4%

---

follow-up of 2.7 years found an independent association between sleep apnea and incident diabetes,[68] the other did not show any association after 4-year follow-up.[69]

OSA may not only increase the risk of dysfunction in glucose metabolism, but also affect glycemic control in patients who already have diabetes. There is a suggestion that OSA severity may play a role in conferring the degree of dysfunction. In an observational cross-sectional study of 52 patients, increased hemoglobin A1C (HbA1c) levels were associated with increased severity.[70] This was independent of age, gender, BMI, duration of diabetes, and insulin dose; however, a plateau effect was noted from moderate to severe OSA levels.

Intermittent hypoxemia and recurrent arousals from sleep are thought to play an important role in pathophysiologic mechanisms leading to altered glucose homeostasis in patients with OSA (**Fig. 3**). Both mice and human studies have shown diminished insulin sensitivity after exposure to intermittent hypoxemia.[71–73] Patients with OSA have elevated blood levels of leptin, an appetite-suppressing adipokine secreted by adipose tissues, largely contributed by oxygen desaturations during sleep.[74,75] Prolonged hyperleptinemia may lead to leptin resistance.[10,76] Patients with OSA also have elevated circulating inflammatory cytokines, such as tumor necrosis factor-alpha and interleukin-6.[77,78] The other 2 possible mechanisms are thought to be activation of the sympathetic nervous system, which can cause upregulation of regulatory factors that have anti-insulin activities, and dysfunction of the hypothalamic-hypophyseal-adrenal axis, which can increase cortisol levels. All of these may contribute to insulin resistance.[10,13,79]

If OSA is associated with insulin resistance, then treatment is expected to improve insulin sensitivity. Nonrandomized trials using CPAP therapy for treating OSA have shown improvement in insulin sensitivity, sleeping glucose levels, and HbA1C, especially in nonobese and nondiabetic patients with OSA.[80–82] The duration of CPAP therapy and the hours of usage per night seem to affect the outcome. The insulin sensitivity improved within 2 days of initiating CPAP therapy in nondiabetic patients who were also not obese, but improvement at 3 months also was seen in patients

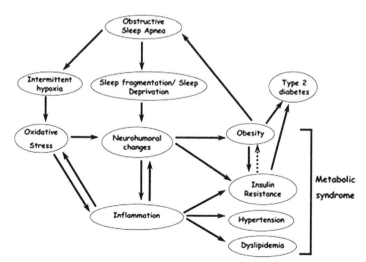

Fig. 3. Possible mechanistic links between OSA, DM2, and metabolic syndrome. Dyslipidemia includes both hypertriglyceridemia and low HDL-cholesterol. (*Reproduced from* Tasali E, Ip MS. Obstructive sleep apnea and metabolic syndrome: alterations in glucose metabolism and inflammation. Proc Am Thorac Soc 2008;5:212; with permission.)

with diabetes irrespective of weight.[80,83] Likewise, a progressive improvement in HbA1C was seen over time with CPAP therapy, but only when CPAP was used for more than 4 hours per night[81]; however, a placebo-controlled CPAP trial did not show any significant improvement in HbA1C and insulin resistance in obese patients with DM2.[84] There is indeed a need for larger controlled trials of longer duration of follow-up to study long-term effects of therapy on glucose metabolism.

METABOLIC SYNDROME

Metabolic syndrome is a constellation of risk factors that are metabolic disturbances in themselves, and predicts an increased risk for future DM2 and cardiovascular diseases. The National Cholesterol Education Program Adult Treatment Panel III has developed criteria consisting of 5 variables (abdominal obesity, triglycerides, high-density lipoprotein cholesterol, blood pressure, and fasting glucose) with set threshold values.[85,86] The presence of 3 or more variables out of 5 qualifies for the diagnosis of metabolic syndrome (**Box 3**). It is hard not to notice that some of the variables, such as obesity, alteration in glucose homeostasis, and hypertension, are associated with OSA as well. In fact, studies have shown that OSA is independently associated with metabolic syndrome,[65,87,88] and that unrecognized OSA is common in patients with metabolic syndrome.[89] Chronic intermittent hypoxemia and sleep fragmentation, as discussed previously, are thought to be involved in the overall pathophysiology (see **Fig. 3**). There is some evidence of OSA therapy improving some of the individual parameters that comprise metabolic syndrome and are discussed elsewhere in this article, but data are scant on the effect of treatment on the whole metabolic syndrome entity and its cardiovascular and diabetic consequences. One study that followed 89 subjects for a period of 12 to 32 months found that metabolic syndrome did not increase the risk of cardiovascular events in CPAP-treated patients with OSA.[90]

GASTROESOPHAGEAL REFLUX DISEASE

During sleep, swallowing frequency decreases and production of saliva ceases. This leads to impaired esophageal acid clearance, thereby increasing acid-mucosa contact time. Gastroesophageal reflux commonly occurs and is noted in sleep as well, and occurs more frequently in patients with gastroesophageal reflux disease. Nocturnal reflux symptoms are increased in patients with OSA.[91] The pathophysiology of this association is not clearly understood, although the pressure gradient across the lower esophageal sphincter that develops during the upper airway collapse is thought to favor reflux. CPAP therapy has been shown to improve not only reflux symptoms in

---

Box 3
Metabolic syndrome criteria: 3 or more variables out of 5 qualify for the diagnosis of metabolic syndrome

- Waist circumference >40 inches in men and 35 inches in women
- Serum triglycerides level $\geq$150 mg/dL
- Serum high-density lipoprotein cholesterol level <40 mg/dL in men and <50 mg/dL in women
- Blood pressure $\geq$130/85 mm Hg
- Fasting glucose level $\geq$100 mg/dL

patients with and without OSA, but also has been shown to improve lower esophageal sphincter function.[92,93]

REFERENCES

1. Lopez-Jimenez F, Sert Kuniyoshi FH, Gami A, et al. Obstructive sleep apnea: implications for cardiac and vascular disease. Chest 2008;133(3):793–804.
2. Lavie L, Lavie P. Molecular mechanisms of cardiovascular disease in OSAHS: the oxidative stress link. Eur Respir J 2009;33(6):1467–84.
3. Somers VK, Dyken ME, Clary MP, et al. Sympathetic neural mechanisms in obstructive sleep apnea. J Clin Invest 1995;96(4):1897–904.
4. Shamsuzzaman AS, Winnicki M, Lanfranchi P, et al. Elevated C-reactive protein in patients with obstructive sleep apnea. Circulation 2002;105(21):2462–4.
5. Punjabi NM, Beamer BA. C-reactive protein is associated with sleep disordered breathing independent of adiposity. Sleep 2007;30(1):29–34.
6. Somers VK, White DP, Amin R, et al. Sleep apnea and cardiovascular disease: an American Heart Association/American College of Cardiology Foundation Scientific Statement from the American Heart Association Council for High Blood Pressure Research Professional Education Committee, Council on Clinical Cardiology, Stroke Council, and Council on Cardiovascular Nursing. J Am Coll Cardiol 2008; 52(8):686–717.
7. von Kanel R, Dimsdale JE. Hemostatic alterations in patients with obstructive sleep apnea and the implications for cardiovascular disease. Chest 2003; 124(5):1956–67.
8. Otto ME, Belohlavek M, Romero-Corral A, et al. Comparison of cardiac structural and functional changes in obese otherwise healthy adults with versus without obstructive sleep apnea. Am J Cardiol 2007;99(9):1298–302.
9. Romero-Corral A, Somers VK, Pellikka PA, et al. Decreased right and left ventricular myocardial performance in obstructive sleep apnea. Chest 2007;132(6): 1863–70.
10. Phillips BG, Kato M, Narkiewicz K, et al. Increases in leptin levels, sympathetic drive, and weight gain in obstructive sleep apnea. Am J Physiol Heart Circ Physiol 2000;279(1):H234–7.
11. Elmasry A, Lindberg E, Berne C, et al. Sleep-disordered breathing and glucose metabolism in hypertensive men: a population-based study. J Intern Med 2001; 249(2):153–61.
12. Punjabi NM, Shahar E, Redline S, et al. Sleep-disordered breathing, glucose intolerance, and insulin resistance: the Sleep Heart Health Study. Am J Epidemiol 2004;160(6):521–30.
13. Punjabi NM, Polotsky VY. Disorders of glucose metabolism in sleep apnea. J Appl Physiol 2005;99(5):1998–2007.
14. Peppard PE, Young T, Palta M, et al. Prospective study of the association between sleep-disordered breathing and hypertension. N Engl J Med 2000; 342(19):1378–84.
15. O'Connor GT, Caffo B, Newman AB, et al. Prospective study of sleep-disordered breathing and hypertension: the Sleep Heart Health Study. Am J Respir Crit Care Med 2009;179(12):1159–64.
16. Peppard PE. Is obstructive sleep apnea a risk factor for hypertension? Differences between the Wisconsin Sleep Cohort and the Sleep Heart Health Study. J Clin Sleep Med 2009;5(5):404–5.

17. Chobanian AV, Bakris GL, Black HR, et al. Seventh report of the Joint National Committee on Prevention, Detection, Evaluation, and Treatment of High Blood Pressure. Hypertension 2003;42(6):1206–52.

18. Ramar K, Caples SM. Vascular changes, cardiovascular disease and obstructive sleep apnea. Future Cardiol 2011;7(2):241–9.

19. Calhoun DA. Obstructive sleep apnea and hypertension. Curr Hypertens Rep 2010;12(3):189–95.

20. Dudenbostel T, Calhoun DA. Resistant hypertension, obstructive sleep apnoea and aldosterone. J Hum Hypertens 2011. [Epub ahead of print].

21. Penzel T, Riedl M, Gapelyuk A, et al. Effect of CPAP therapy on daytime cardiovascular regulations in patients with obstructive sleep apnea. Comput Biol Med 2012;42(3):328–34.

22. Buchner NJ, Quack I, Stegbauer J, et al. Treatment of obstructive sleep apnea reduces arterial stiffness. Sleep Breath 2012;16(1):123–33.

23. Andren A, Sjoquist M, Tegelberg A. Effects on blood pressure after treatment of obstructive sleep apnoea with a mandibular advancement appliance—a three-year follow-up. J Oral Rehabil 2009;36(10):719–25.

24. Otsuka R, Ribeiro de Almeida F, Lowe AA, et al. The effect of oral appliance therapy on blood pressure in patients with obstructive sleep apnea. Sleep Breath 2006;10(1):29–36.

25. Kohler M, Stradling JR. Mechanisms of vascular damage in obstructive sleep apnea. Nat Rev Cardiol 2010;7(12):677–85.

26. Alonso-Fernandez A, Garcia-Rio F, Racionero MA, et al. Cardiac rhythm disturbances and ST-segment depression episodes in patients with obstructive sleep apnea-hypopnea syndrome and its mechanisms. Chest 2005;127(1):15–22.

27. Peker Y, Hedner J, Norum J, et al. Increased incidence of cardiovascular disease in middle-aged men with obstructive sleep apnea: a 7-year follow-up. Am J Respir Crit Care Med 2002;166(2):159–65.

28. Marin JM, Carrizo SJ, Vicente E, et al. Long-term cardiovascular outcomes in men with obstructive sleep apnoea-hypopnoea with or without treatment with continuous positive airway pressure: an observational study. Lancet 2005;365(9464):1046–53.

29. Peled N, Abinader EG, Pillar G, et al. Nocturnal ischemic events in patients with obstructive sleep apnea syndrome and ischemic heart disease: effects of continuous positive air pressure treatment. J Am Coll Cardiol 1999;34(6):1744–9.

30. Gami AS, Svatikova A, Wolk R, et al. Cardiac troponin T in obstructive sleep apnea. Chest 2004;125(6):2097–100.

31. Colish J, Walker JR, Elmayergi N, et al. Obstructive sleep apnea: effects of continuous positive airway pressure on cardiac remodeling as assessed by cardiac biomarkers, echocardiography, and cardiac MRI. Chest 2011. [Epub ahead of print].

32. Olmetti F, La Rovere MT, Robbi E, et al. Nocturnal cardiac arrhythmia in patients with obstructive sleep apnea. Sleep Med 2008;9(5):475–80.

33. Hoffstein V, Mateika S. Cardiac arrhythmias, snoring, and sleep apnea. Chest 1994;106(2):466–71.

34. Hanak V, Konecny T, Somers VK. Cardiovascular pathophysiology of sleep apnea. In: Avidan AY, Barkoukis TJ, editors. Review of sleep medicine. 3rd edition. Philadelphia: Elsevier-Saunders; 2011. p. 143–50.

35. Kanagala R, Murali NS, Friedman PA, et al. Obstructive sleep apnea and the recurrence of atrial fibrillation. Circulation 2003;107(20):2589–94.

36. Ng CY, Liu T, Shehata M, et al. Meta-analysis of obstructive sleep apnea as predictor of atrial fibrillation recurrence after catheter ablation. Am J Cardiol 2011;108(1):47–51.
37. Sajkov D, McEvoy RD. Obstructive sleep apnea and pulmonary hypertension. Prog Cardiovasc Dis 2009;51(5):363–70.
38. Sajkov D, Wang T, Saunders NA, et al. Daytime pulmonary hemodynamics in patients with obstructive sleep apnea without lung disease. Am J Respir Crit Care Med 1999;159(5 Pt 1):1518–26.
39. Easton JD, Saver JL, Albers GW, et al. Definition and evaluation of transient ischemic attack: a scientific statement for healthcare professionals from the American Heart Association/American Stroke Association Stroke Council; Council on Cardiovascular Surgery and Anesthesia; Council on Cardiovascular Radiology and Intervention; Council on Cardiovascular Nursing; and the Interdisciplinary Council on Peripheral Vascular Disease. The American Academy of Neurology affirms the value of this statement as an educational tool for neurologists. Stroke 2009;40(6):2276–93.
40. Roger VL, Go AS, Lloyd-Jones DM, et al. Heart disease and stroke statistics—2011 update: a report from the American Heart Association. Circulation 2011;123(4):e18–209.
41. Smirne S, Palazzi S, Zucconi M, et al. Habitual snoring as a risk factor for acute vascular disease. Eur Respir J 1993;6(9):1357–61.
42. Yaggi HK, Concato J, Kernan WN, et al. Obstructive sleep apnea as a risk factor for stroke and death. N Engl J Med 2005;353(19):2034–41.
43. Sanner BM, Konermann M, Tepel M, et al. Platelet function in patients with obstructive sleep apnoea syndrome. Eur Respir J 2000;16(4):648–52.
44. Ip MS, Tse HF, Lam B, et al. Endothelial function in obstructive sleep apnea and response to treatment. Am J Respir Crit Care Med 2004;169(3):348–53.
45. Lee SA, Amis TC, Byth K, et al. Heavy snoring as a cause of carotid artery atherosclerosis. Sleep 2008;31(9):1207–13.
46. Suzuki T, Nakano H, Maekawa J, et al. Obstructive sleep apnea and carotid-artery intima-media thickness. Sleep 2004;27(1):129–33.
47. Hermann DM, Bassetti CL. Sleep-related breathing and sleep-wake disturbances in ischemic stroke. Neurology 2009;73(16):1313–22.
48. Parra O, Arboix A, Bechich S, et al. Time course of sleep-related breathing disorders in first-ever stroke or transient ischemic attack. Am J Respir Crit Care Med 2000;161(2 Pt 1):375–80.
49. Good DC, Henkle JQ, Gelber D, et al. Sleep-disordered breathing and poor functional outcome after stroke. Stroke 1996;27(2):252–9.
50. Sahlin C, Sandberg O, Gustafson Y, et al. Obstructive sleep apnea is a risk factor for death in patients with stroke: a 10-year follow-up. Arch Intern Med 2008;168(3):297–301.
51. Martinez-Garcia MA, Galiano-Blancart R, Roman-Sanchez P, et al. Continuous positive airway pressure treatment in sleep apnea prevents new vascular events after ischemic stroke. Chest 2005;128(4):2123–9.
52. Sandberg O, Franklin KA, Bucht G, et al. Nasal continuous positive airway pressure in stroke patients with sleep apnoea: a randomized treatment study. Eur Respir J 2001;18(4):630–4.
53. Association AD. Diagnosis and classification of diabetes mellitus. Diabetes Care 2011;34(Suppl 1):s62–9.
54. Genuth S, Alberti KG, Bennett P, et al. Follow-up report on the diagnosis of diabetes mellitus. Diabetes Care 2003;26(11):3160–7.

55. Makino S, Handa H, Suzukawa K, et al. Obstructive sleep apnoea syndrome, plasma adiponectin levels, and insulin resistance. Clin Endocrinol (Oxf) 2006; 64(1):12–9.

56. Kono M, Tatsumi K, Saibara T, et al. Obstructive sleep apnea syndrome is associated with some components of metabolic syndrome. Chest 2007;131(5): 1387–92.

57. McArdle N, Hillman D, Beilin L, et al. Metabolic risk factors for vascular disease in obstructive sleep apnea: a matched controlled study. Am J Respir Crit Care Med 2007;175(2):190–5.

58. Meslier N, Gagnadoux F, Giraud P, et al. Impaired glucose-insulin metabolism in males with obstructive sleep apnoea syndrome. Eur Respir J 2003;22(1): 156–60.

59. Grunstein RR, Stenlof K, Hedner J, et al. Impact of obstructive sleep apnea and sleepiness on metabolic and cardiovascular risk factors in the Swedish Obese Subjects (SOS) Study. Int J Obes Relat Metab Disord 1995;19(6):410–8.

60. Jennum P, Schultz-Larsen K, Christensen N. Snoring, sympathetic activity and cardiovascular risk factors in a 70 year old population. Eur J Epidemiol 1993; 9(5):477–82.

61. Renko AK, Hiltunen L, Laakso M, et al. The relationship of glucose tolerance to sleep disorders and daytime sleepiness. Diabetes Res Clin Pract 2005;67(1): 84–91.

62. Joo S, Lee S, Choi HA, et al. Habitual snoring is associated with elevated hemoglobin A1c levels in non-obese middle-aged adults. J Sleep Res 2006;15(4): 437–44.

63. Thomas GN, Jiang CQ, Lao XQ, et al. Snoring and vascular risk factors and disease in a low-risk Chinese population: the Guangzhou Biobank Cohort Study. Sleep 2006;29(7):896–900.

64. Okada M, Takamizawa A, Tsushima K, et al. Relationship between sleep-disordered breathing and lifestyle-related illnesses in subjects who have undergone health-screening. Intern Med 2006;45(15):891–6.

65. Lam JC, Lam B, Lam CL, et al. Obstructive sleep apnea and the metabolic syndrome in community-based Chinese adults in Hong Kong. Respir Med 2006;100(6):980–7.

66. Elmasry A, Janson C, Lindberg E, et al. The role of habitual snoring and obesity in the development of diabetes: a 10-year follow-up study in a male population. J Intern Med 2000;248(1):13–20.

67. Al-Delaimy WK, Manson JE, Willett WC, et al. Snoring as a risk factor for type II diabetes mellitus: a prospective study. Am J Epidemiol 2002;155(5):387–93.

68. Botros N, Concato J, Mohsenin V, et al. Obstructive sleep apnea as a risk factor for type 2 diabetes. Am J Med 2009;122(12):1122–7.

69. Reichmuth KJ, Austin D, Skatrud JB, et al. Association of sleep apnea and type II diabetes: a population-based study. Am J Respir Crit Care Med 2005;172(12): 1590–5.

70. Pillai A, Warren G, Gunathilake W, et al. Effects of sleep apnea severity on glycemic control in patients with type 2 diabetes prior to continuous positive airway pressure treatment. Diabetes Technol Ther 2011;13(9):945–9.

71. Iiyori N, Alonso LC, Li J, et al. Intermittent hypoxia causes insulin resistance in lean mice independent of autonomic activity. Am J Respir Crit Care Med 2007; 175(8):851–7.

72. Polotsky VY, Li J, Punjabi NM, et al. Intermittent hypoxia increases insulin resistance in genetically obese mice. J Physiol 2003;552(Pt 1):253–64.

73. Louis M, Punjabi NM. Effects of acute intermittent hypoxia on glucose metabolism in awake healthy volunteers. J Appl Physiol 2009;106(5):1538–44.
74. Tatsumi K, Kasahara Y, Kurosu K, et al. Sleep oxygen desaturation and circulating leptin in obstructive sleep apnea-hypopnea syndrome. Chest 2005;127(3):716–21.
75. Chin K, Shimizu K, Nakamura T, et al. Changes in intra-abdominal visceral fat and serum leptin levels in patients with obstructive sleep apnea syndrome following nasal continuous positive airway pressure therapy. Circulation 1999;100(7): 706–12.
76. Considine RV, Sinha MK, Heiman ML, et al. Serum immunoreactive-leptin concentrations in normal-weight and obese humans. N Engl J Med 1996;334(5):292–5.
77. Ryan S, Taylor CT, McNicholas WT. Selective activation of inflammatory pathways by intermittent hypoxia in obstructive sleep apnea syndrome. Circulation 2005; 112(17):2660–7.
78. Garvey JF, Taylor CT, McNicholas WT. Cardiovascular disease in obstructive sleep apnoea syndrome: the role of intermittent hypoxia and inflammation. Eur Respir J 2009;33(5):1195–205.
79. Polotsky VY, Jun J, Punjabi NM. Obstructive sleep apnea and metabolic dysfunction. In: Kryger MH, Roth T, Dement WC, editors. Principles and practice of sleep medicine. 5th edition. St Louis (MO): Elsevier Saunders; 2011. p. 1331–8.
80. Harsch IA, Schahin SP, Radespiel-Troger M, et al. Continuous positive airway pressure treatment rapidly improves insulin sensitivity in patients with obstructive sleep apnea syndrome. Am J Respir Crit Care Med 2004;169(2):156–62.
81. Babu AR, Herdegen J, Fogelfeld L, et al. Type 2 diabetes, glycemic control, and continuous positive airway pressure in obstructive sleep apnea. Arch Intern Med 2005;165(4):447–52.
82. Dawson A, Abel SL, Loving RT, et al. CPAP therapy of obstructive sleep apnea in type 2 diabetics improves glycemic control during sleep. J Clin Sleep Med 2008; 4(6):538–42.
83. Harsch IA, Schahin SP, Bruckner K, et al. The effect of continuous positive airway pressure treatment on insulin sensitivity in patients with obstructive sleep apnoea syndrome and type 2 diabetes. Respiration 2004;71(3):252–9.
84. West SD, Nicoll DJ, Wallace TM, et al. Effect of CPAP on insulin resistance and HbA1c in men with obstructive sleep apnoea and type 2 diabetes. Thorax 2007;62(11):969–74.
85. National Cholesterol Education Program (NCEP) Expert Panel on Detection, Evaluation, and Treatment of High Blood Cholesterol in Adults (Adult Treatment Panel III). Third Report of the National Cholesterol Education Program (NCEP) Expert Panel on Detection, Evaluation, and Treatment of High Blood Cholesterol in Adults (Adult Treatment Panel III) final report. Circulation 2002;106(25):3143–421.
86. Grundy SM, Cleeman JI, Daniels SR, et al. Diagnosis and management of the metabolic syndrome: an American Heart Association/National Heart, Lung, and Blood Institute Scientific Statement. Circulation 2005;112(17):2735–52.
87. Coughlin SR, Mawdsley L, Mugarza JA, et al. Obstructive sleep apnoea is independently associated with an increased prevalence of metabolic syndrome. Eur Heart J 2004;25(9):735–41.
88. Chin K, Oga T, Takahashi K, et al. Associations between obstructive sleep apnea, metabolic syndrome, and sleep duration, as measured with an actigraph, in an urban male working population in Japan. Sleep 2010;33(1):89–95.
89. Drager LF, Lopes HF, Maki-Nunes C, et al. The impact of obstructive sleep apnea on metabolic and inflammatory markers in consecutive patients with metabolic syndrome. PLoS One 2010;5(8):e12065.

90. Ambrosetti M, Lucioni AM, Conti S, et al. Metabolic syndrome in obstructive sleep apnea and related cardiovascular risk. J Cardiovasc Med (Hagerstown) 2006; 7(11):826–9.

91. Shepherd KL, James AL, Musk AW, et al. Gastro-oesophageal reflux symptoms are related to the presence and severity of obstructive sleep apnoea. J Sleep Res 2011;20(1 Pt 2):241–9.

92. Shepherd KL, Holloway RH, Hillman DR, et al. The impact of continuous positive airway pressure on the lower esophageal sphincter. Am J Physiol Gastrointest Liver Physiol 2007;292(5):G1200–5.

93. Orr WC. CPAP and things that go "burp" in the night. J Clin Sleep Med 2008;4(5): 439–40.

94. Gami AS, Howard DE, Olson EJ, et al. Day-night pattern of sudden death in obstructive sleep apnea. N Engl J Med 2005;352(12):1206–14.

Sleep Bruxism: A Comprehensive Overview for the Dental Clinician Interested in Sleep Medicine

Maria Clotilde Carra, DMD*, Nelly Huynh, PhD,
Gilles Lavigne, DMD, PhD, FRDC

KEYWORDS

- Sleep bruxism • Tooth grinding • Tooth clenching
- Sleep arousal • Sleep-disordered breathing • Headache
- Temporomandibular disorders

DEFINITION AND CLASSIFICATION OF SLEEP BRUXISM

In dentistry, bruxism is traditionally considered an oral parafunction characterized by involuntary grinding and clenching of the teeth.[1,2] Although this definition describes the main characteristics of the disorder, it lacks a substantial and important distinction between the wake and sleep states in which this oral parafunction may occur. In fact, a wake-time habit of clenching, grinding, or gnashing the teeth seems to be a different nosologic entity, probably with a different cause and pathophysiology, and it should be distinguished from bruxism during sleep.

According to the American Academy of Sleep Medicine (AASM) (*International Classification of Sleep Disorders, Second Edition* [ICSD-II]),[3] sleep bruxism (SB) is

Disclosure of financial and conflicts of interest: M.C. Carra received a scholarship from the Ministère de l'Éducation, du Loisir et du Sport du Québec. G. Lavigne is a Canada Research Chair, and his research is supported by the Canadian Institutes of Health Research (CIHR grant MOP - 11701), FRSQ, and CFI. He has been an invited speaker, lecturer, or consultant with UCB Belgium, Pfizer (Wyeth) Canada and Medotech (Grindcare), Denmark. The authors' group also receives, free or at reduced cost, oral appliances for research purposes (ORM-Narval, France-Canada; Silencer, Canada; Klearway, Canada) with no obligation attached. N. Huynh declares no financial conflicts of interest.
Faculty of Dental Medicine, Univeristé de Montréal, CP 6128 Succursale Centre-Ville, Montreal, Quebec, H3C 3J7, Canada
* Corresponding author.
E-mail addresses: maria.clotilde.carra@umontreal.ca; mclotildecarra@gmail.com

Dent Clin N Am 56 (2012) 387–413
doi:10.1016/j.cden.2012.01.003
0011-8532/12/$ – see front matter © 2012 Elsevier Inc. All rights reserved.

classified as a sleep-related movement disorder. The characteristic electromyography (EMG) pattern of SB is found in repetitive and recurrent episodes of rhythmic masticatory muscle activity (RMMA) of the masseter and temporalis muscles that are usually associated with sleep arousals.[3,4] RMMA shows a frequency of 1 Hz and typically occurs cyclically during sleep (**Fig. 1**).[4] RMMA episodes are observed in 60% of the general adult population as physiologic activity of the jaw muscles during sleep.[5,6] Many other forms of masticatory and facial muscle activity are also observed during sleep, such as swallowing, coughing, sleep talking, smiling, lip sucking, jaw movements, and myoclonus.[4,7] These orofacial activities account for approximately 85% of EMG events scored on the masseter and temporalis muscles in control subjects and 30% in patients with SB.[5,8–10] In fact, RMMA frequency is 3 times higher in patients with SB than in controls and is typically associated with tooth-grinding sounds (in 45% of cases), as reported by patients, bed partners, parents, or siblings.

SB may be an extreme manifestation of a physiologic orofacial motor behavior during sleep (RMMA and chewinglike activity) whereby certain factors increase its occurrence until it falls into the pathologic range of jaw-muscle activity.[11,12] Therefore, SB refers to the sleep motor disorder, whereas RMMA is the characteristic EMG pattern that is scored during sleep to make a polysomnographic diagnosis of SB.

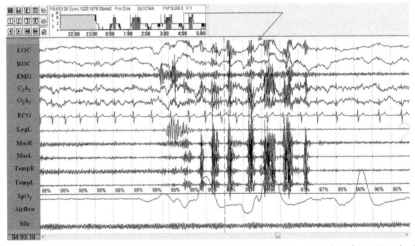

Fig. 1. Hypnogram and polysomnographic tracing showing an episode of RMMA during sleep. The full-night hypnogram (graph in the upper left) represents sleep stage distribution in non-REM sleep 1, 2, 3, 4, and REM sleep, whereas the 20-second polysomnographic page shows a clear example of RMMA during sleep. The patient is in non-REM sleep stage 2. RMMA is defined when at least 3 consecutive EMG bursts (frequency 1 Hz) lasting greater than or equal to 0.25 seconds are scored on the masseter and temporalis channels. Corresponding with the RMMA episode, note the increased frequency in cortical activity (EEG central [C_3A_2] and occipital [O_1A_2] derivations), increased heart rate (on the ECG channel), and increased amplitude of respiratory airflow (naso-cannula). Immediately before the RMMA onset, a leg movement event is also seen on the EMG channel of the tibialis muscle. Airflow, naso-cannula airflow; C_3A_2, the central derivation of the electroencephalogram; ECG, electrocardiogram; EMG, electromyographic activity of the suprahyoid muscle; LOC, left electrooculogram; LegL, EMG of the left tibialis muscle; MasR and MasL, EMG of the right and left masseter muscles; Mic, microphone; O_1A_2, the occipital derivation of the EEG; ROC, right electrooculogram; SpO2, oxygen saturation level (expressed as %); TempR and TempL, EMG of the right and left temporalis muscles.

ASSESSMENT AND DIAGNOSIS OF SB

The assessment and diagnosis of SB are often challenging. Generally, the assessment is based on reports of tooth-grinding sounds during sleep and the presence of clinical signs and symptoms.[3] However, only an EMG recording of the masticatory muscles can confirm the SB diagnosis. Several portable diagnostic tools have been developed to record masseter or temporalis EMG activity during sleep to avoid using the more sophisticated but highly cost- and time-consuming polysomnography (PSG). However, the reliability of most portable devices has not yet been validated, and their use may be considered only as support in a clinical assessment of SB. In fact, the SB diagnosis is usually clinical, although the gold standard remains a full-night PSG with audio-video recording (**Table 1**). The future direction for SB assessment would be to develop a handy tool that can directly, reliably, and rapidly measure ongoing bruxism activity and that can be used in both clinical (for diagnosis, treatment outcome evaluation, and follow-up) and research settings.

Clinical Diagnosis of SB

The clinical diagnosis of SB should be based on the international diagnostic criteria proposed by the AASM (**Box 1**).[3,13] Grinding sounds caused by tooth contacts are the pathognomonic sign of SB and they are usually reported by patients, bed partners, siblings, or parents. However, not all RMMA episodes are accompanied by tooth grinding and many patients or family members may not be aware of this.

A clinical examination of the oral cavity allows identifying signs and symptoms that are markers of tooth-grinding activity and a clenching habit. These signs and symptoms include hypertrophy of the masseter and temporalis muscles, tongue indentation, tooth wear, jaw muscle tenderness or pain on digital palpation, and reports of morning headache.[4,14] However, none of these signs and symptoms constitutes direct proof of current SB activity. For example, although tooth wear is widely reported in the literature as the classic dental sign of bruxism (both awake and during sleep), it may be related to many other factors that can induce attrition and erosion on dental surfaces (eg, age, occlusal conditions, enamel characteristics, diet, carbonated drinks, medications, gastroesophageal reflux, and alimentary disorders).[4,14–18] Moreover, it was recently demonstrated that tooth wear cannot be used as an absolute criterion to assess SB severity: no difference in tooth wear grade was found between low and high frequency of muscle contractions in young adults with SB.[16]

During the clinical examination, dental clinicians can also identify early risk factors for SB and other sleep or medical disorders (eg, sleep-disordered breathing) and promote further investigations when necessary. In particular, the risk of having or developing sleep-disordered breathing (SDB) increases with retrognathia, micrognathia, macroglossia, adenotonsillar hypertrophy, and a Mallampati score of III and IV.[19] The Mallampati score qualifies oropharyngeal obstruction, with I standing for no obstruction (tonsils, pillars, and soft palate are clearly visible) and IV for high obstruction (only the hard palate is visible).[20] In addition, clinicians can directly observe breathing habits (mouth breathing vs nasal breathing), behavioral attitudes (agitation, anxiety), and a tendency to fall asleep. Although it remains under investigation, some of these factors have been associated with an increased risk for both SB and SDB.[21]

Appropriate questionnaires can also be used to investigate general health, quality of life, pain, headache, sleep quality, and sleepiness. Some questionnaires have been validated for both clinical and research purposes (eg, the Pittsburg Sleep Quality Index and the Epworth Sleepiness Scale). Questionnaire assessments may give the clinician

Table 1
Methods for assessing SB (order of increasing reliability)

Method	Notes
Patient history	Many patients may not be aware of their tooth-grinding habit during sleep. It is more reliable if the bed partner, parents, or siblings report current tooth-grinding sounds during sleep
Clinical assessment	It is used to assess the clinical signs and symptoms that suggest SB (eg, tooth wear; see **Box 1**) and the presence of potential risk factors for other comorbidities (eg, enlarged tonsils, skeletal class II, and Mallampati score III or IV for the risk of concomitant SDB)
Questionnaires	It is used to investigate patients' general and oral health, sleep quality, sleep habits, oral parafunctions, presence and characteristics of pain, headache, fatigue, depression, anxiety and stress, and comorbidities.
Ambulatory EMG monitoring	It allows recording EMG activity during sleep from the temporalis or masseter muscles, depending on the device used. However, there is very low specificity and sensitivity in distinguishing actual RMMA episodes from the many other orofacial and motor activities that occur during sleep. Furthermore, there is no monitoring on awakening from sleep, arousal, sleep staging, or other sleep variables. This tool could be valuable in the clinical assessment of SB and in large-sample studies (eg, general population epidemiologic studies)
Ambulatory PSG recording (type II, III, and IV)	It is usually performed at patients' homes. Normally, there is no audio-video monitoring; specificity and sensitivity in detecting RMMA depends on the device used, and more particularly, on the number of variables monitored (EEG, EOG, ECG, EMG, and respiratory channels). This method may be used for scoring sleep stages, sleep arousals, leg movements, and EMG activity, and for monitoring breathing
Full audio-video PSG recording (type I)	It remains the gold standard for the diagnosis of SB and the assessment of comorbidity with other sleep disorders (eg, SDB, PLMS, RLS, RBD, parasomnias). Normally, it allows full-night monitoring of EEG, EOG, EMG, ECG, leg movements, respiratory effort, airflow, and oxygen saturation. Concomitant audio-video recording increases the specificity and sensitivity in RMMA detection and scoring by distinguishing between RMMA episodes and orofacial (eg, swallowing, coughing, sleep talking) and other muscular activities (eg, head movements, eye blinking) that occur during sleep

Abbreviations: ECG, electrocardiogram; EEG, electroencephalogram; EOG, elecrooculogram; PLMS, periodic limb movement during sleep; RBD, REM sleep behavior disorder; RLS, restless leg syndrome; SDB, sleep-disordered breathing.

Data from Lavigne G, Manzini C, Huynh NT. Sleep Bruxism. In: Kryger MH, Roth T, Dement WC, editors. Principles and practice of sleep medicine. 5th edition. St Louis (MO): Elsevier Saunders; 2011. p. 1129–39; and Hirshkowitz M, Kryger MH. Monitoring techniques for evaluating suspected sleep-disordered breathing. In: Kryger MH, Roth T, Dement WC, editors. Principles and practice of sleep medicine. 5th edition. St Louis (MO): Elsevier Saunders; 2011. p. 1610–23.

an indication of the risk of comorbidity between SB and other, more severe sleep disorders, such as SDB or restless leg syndrome (RLS) (see **Table 1**).

Ambulatory Assessment of SB

Several portable EMG monitoring systems have been developed to assess SB activity. They differ in degree of complexity, ranging from miniature self-contained EMG detectors to ambulatory PSG systems (type II, III, and IV),[22] which allow monitoring only a limited number of channels (see **Table 1**). These devices enable multiple-night

---

Box 1
AASM clinical diagnostic criteria for SB

Patient history

- Recent patient, parent, or sibling report of tooth-grinding sounds occurring during sleep for at least 3 to 5 nights per week in the last 3 to 6 months

Clinical evaluation[a]

- Abnormal tooth wear

- Hypertrophy of the masseter muscles on voluntary forceful clenching

- Discomfort, fatigue, or pain in the jaw muscles (and transient, morning jaw-muscle pain and headache)

Jaw-muscle activity cannot be better explained by another current sleep disorder, medical or neurologic disorder, medication use, or substance use disorder.

[a] None of these signs and symptoms constitutes direct proof of current SB activity. Full-night PSG with audio-video recording remains the gold standard for SB diagnosis.
   Data from International classification of sleep disorders, 2nd ed.: Diagnosis and coding manual. (ICSD-2). Westchester, Illinois.: American Academy of Sleep Medicine (AASM) eds.; 2005. Section on Sleep Related Bruxism. p.189–92; and Lavigne G, Manzini C, Huynh NT. Sleep Bruxism. In: Kryger MH, Roth T, Dement WC, editors. Principles and practice of sleep medicine. 5th edition. St Louis (MO): Elsevier Saunders; 2011. p. 1129–39.

---

recordings in patients' homes at minimal expense and could be useful research tools in large sample studies. However, the lack of standardized scoring criteria and evidence-based validity limit their application to both clinical and research settings.

Because automatic EMG detectors and analyzers usually use a unique algorithm for RMMA activity scoring, their validity remains to be demonstrated. Conversely, ambulatory PSG recordings provide very good quality EMG signals and, depending on their complexity, they can usually assess other sleep parameters, such as sleep electroencephalogram (EEG) (essential for sleep staging) or respiratory variables. In addition, on the masseter or temporalis EMG channels, RMMA episodes can be distinguished as phasic, tonic, or mixed. Furthermore, episode and burst frequency and muscular strength can be calculated (**Box 2**).[4] However, ambulatory PSG is usually performed in the patients' homes without audio-video monitoring. This situation may lead to the overestimation of RMMA episodes because of confounding and non-SB–specific motor activities during sleep. The authors are currently validating RMMA scoring criteria on ambulatory PSG recordings and have observed a modest concordance rate between RMMA scored with and without video on the same night (Carra, unpublished data, 2012). Although preliminary, this finding suggests that, in the absence of audio-video recording, more rigorous criteria should be applied to the clinical assessment and EMG scoring of SB-related activity.

Polysomnographic Diagnosis of SB

PSG for SB is mainly used for research purposes (see **Table 1**). The research diagnostic criteria have been developed from PSG with audio-video recordings performed in a hospital setting with a sleep technician attending full-night monitoring.[9,13] This PSG (referred to as type I)[22] allows assessing several sleep physiologic parameters (eg, EEG, electrooculogram, electromyogram, electrocardiogram, airflow, respiratory effort, oxygen saturation), whereas audio-video recording enables documenting tooth-grinding sounds and distinguishing between RMMA and orofacial (eg,

---

Box 2
Polysomnographic research diagnostic criteria for SB for scoring RMMA episodes

Mean EMG amplitude: at least 10% of maximum voluntary clenching activity

Types of RMMA episodes

- PHASIC: at least 3 EMG bursts lasting $\geq$0.25 seconds and <2 seconds
- TONIC: 1 EMG burst lasting >2 seconds
- MIXED: phasic and tonic bursts
- EMG bursts must be separated by <2 seconds to be considered part of the same episode.

SB diagnosis can be made based on[a]

- The RMMA INDEX: number of RMMA episodes per hour of sleep
- The BURST INDEX: number of EMG bursts per hour of sleep
- The BRUXISM TIME INDEX (%): total time spent bruxing/total sleep time $\times$ 100
- TOOTH-GRINDING SOUNDS: at least 1 RMMA episode with tooth-grinding sounds

Positive SB diagnosis (based on the frequency of EMG episodes with positive tooth-grinding history or confirmation in a sleep laboratory)[a]

- LOW FREQUENCY: when the RMMA index $\geq$2 and <4
- HIGH FREQUENCY: when the RMMA index is $\geq$4 or the burst index $\geq$25

[a] Best level of reliability when performing audio-video PSG recordings and the presence of at least 2 RMMA episodes associated with tooth-grinding sounds.
  Data from Refs.[3,4,9,23–26]

---

swallowing) and other muscular activity (eg, head movements) during sleep. The validated criteria for a sleep laboratory diagnosis of SB showed 72% sensitivity and 94% specificity.[9] Based on the RMMA index (number of episodes per hour of sleep), SB is diagnosed when RMMA episodes are greater than or equal to 2 (low-frequency SB, mild bruxism) or RMMA episodes are greater than or equal to 4 (high-frequency SB, severe bruxism) (see **Box 2**).[4,9,27]

PSG recordings are not usually indicated for patients who report SB only. However, the clinician should refer patients to a sleep physician for further investigation and diagnosis if other sleep disorders are suspected (eg, sleep apnea, sleep-related epilepsy, rapid eye movement [REM] sleep behavior disorder, periodic limb movement, or other neurologic disorder).

EPIDEMIOLOGY OF SB

In large population-based studies, it is difficult to assess SB by objective measures, such as PSG recordings. The epidemiology of SB is, therefore, largely determined by questionnaires, self-reports, or clinical findings (eg, tooth wear).

SB is reported by 8% of the general adult population.[28,29] It typically peaks during childhood (with prevalence approaching 40% in children aged less than 11 years)[30–36] and tends to decrease after adulthood. No gender difference has been observed.[28,29,34,37] SB is a common sleep disorder. However, the wide prevalence range reported in the literature is most probably because many studies failed to distinguish between wake-time and sleep-related bruxism or to assess the presence of medical comorbidities that may influence its occurrence. Indeed, SB is frequently concomitant (approximately one-third of patients) with wake-time bruxism, which is characterized mainly by a tooth-clenching habit.[38] Wake-time bruxism tends to increase with age, with an estimated prevalence of 12% in children[21,32] and more than 20% in adults.[32,39–41]

CAUSE AND PATHOGENESIS OF SB

The exact cause and pathophysiology of SB are still unknown.[42] The putative etiologic mechanisms for SB genesis include sleep arousal, autonomic sympathetic-cardiac activation, genetic predisposition, neurochemicals, psychosocial components, exogenous factors, and comorbidities (**Table 2**).

Masticatory muscle movements during sleep (RMMA) are probably different from chewing activity while awake. In fact, SB is characterized by rhythmic motor activity

Table 2
Cause and pathophysiology of SB

Putative Etiologic Factors and Mechanisms	Evidence[a]
Sleep arousal More than 80% of RMMA episodes occur in association with sleep arousal. However, sleep arousal is considered the permissive window that facilitates RMMA occurrence during sleep rather than a trigger or cause of SB	+++
Autonomic sympathetic cardiac activity An increase in sympathetic cardiac activity precedes the onset of most RMMA episodes. This increase is also followed by an increase in heart rate and blood pressure immediately before the muscular activity of the jaw opening and closing muscles	+++
Neurochemicals The potential role of catecholamines (adrenaline, noradrenalin, and dopamine); Patients with SB seem to have higher urinary levels of catecholamines. The putative role of other neurochemicals includes: gamma-aminobutyric acid, orexin, serotonin, and acetylcholine (all involved in the genesis and maintenance of wake and sleep; as yet unknown roles)	+
Genetic and familial predisposition In more than 80% of cases, SB persists from childhood to adulthood. Higher concordance in monozygotic than dizygotic twins. Approximately one-third of patients with SB have a direct family member with a positive tooth grinding history	+
Psychosocial factors Anxiety and stress are risk factors for SB. Patients with SB seem to have maladaptive coping strategies and a more task-oriented personality than patients without SB.	++
Exogenous factors Alcohol, caffeine, cigarette smoking, illicit drug use (eg, cocaine, ecstasy), and medication intake (eg, SSRI) can trigger or increase wake-time bruxism and SB activity	++
Comorbidity A common underlying pathogenetic mechanism is suspected (eg, SB and SDB: does SB play a role in reinstating airway patency following an apnea event, or is SB an apnea-related arousal reaction?)	++

Abbreviation: SSRI, selective serotonin reuptake inhibitor.
  +, weak evidence; ++, moderate evidence; +++, strong evidence.
  [a] Strength of available scientific evidence.
  Data from Refs.[4,15,42,44,48,52,58,70,72,76,78,99,114]

that occurs without any food triturating purpose and is associated with co-contraction of both the jaw-closing and jaw-opening muscles. Moreover, although SB occurs without apparent cortical involvement, unlike chewing, which is initiated at the cortical level, it is strongly influenced by autonomic nervous system activity and arousals during sleep.[15,43] Nevertheless, many scientific studies suggest that SB is centrally regulated, probably in the brainstem, and its genesis is more likely multifactorial.[4,44–46] Conversely, there is little scientific evidence to support a predominant role for peripheral factors, such as occlusal interferences, in the cause of SB.[47]

Sleep Arousal

According to the ICSD-II definition, most RMMA episodes (75%–88%) occur in association with sleep arousals.[3,13,48] This association was first observed by Reding and colleagues[49] in 1968 and by Satoh and Harada[50] in 1971, who described tooth-grinding activity as an arousal reaction. Since then, many studies have used polysom-nography and electrophysiology to investigate the complex relationship between SB and sleep arousal.[11,12,42,48,51–53] Sleep arousal is defined as a brief awakening from sleep (for at least 3 seconds) characterized by increased EEG, autonomic, cardiac, and muscular activities without a complete return to consciousness.[13] Arousals nor-mally reoccur from 6 to 14 times per hour of sleep as the response of the sleeping brain to external (environmental) and internal (physiologic or pathologic) stimuli. Recent evidence on the pathophysiology of SB supports the hypothesis that the frequency of RMMA episodes is modulated by the cyclic occurrence of sleep arousals, called the cyclic alternating pattern (CAP).[12,42,48,49,52] CAP is scored on non-REM sleep EEG to identify periods of stable sleep (phase B) that alternate with periods of active and unstable sleep (phase A, arousal).[54,55]

RMMA episodes are observed more frequently in non-REM sleep stages 1 and 2 (light sleep), in sleep stage shifts, and especially in the transition period from non-REM to REM sleep.[4,48,52,56] More than 80% of RMMA episodes are time correlated with CAP phase A, and they recur in rhythmic clusters, with a periodicity of 20 to 30 seconds, which is similar to the physiologic arousal rhythm of CAP.[12,48,52] Notwith-standing this strong association between sleep arousal and SB, sleep arousals (and CAP phase A) are neither the cause nor the trigger of SB. Instead, they constitute the permissive window that facilitates RMMA during sleep.[12,56]

Autonomic Sympathetic-Cardiac Activity

Recent evidence on SB pathophysiology highlights the role of the autonomic nervous system.[42,46,57] It has been well demonstrated that RMMA onset is associated with a sequence of physiologic events that occur within a sleep arousal. Briefly, the genesis of most RMMA episodes is preceded by the following cascade of events[4]:

- An increase in the autonomic sympathetic-cardiac activity with a concomitant with-drawal of parasympathetic influences (from 8 to 4 minutes before RMMA onset)[52]
- The appearance of rapid-frequency EEG cortical activity (sleep arousal; approx-imately 4 seconds before RMMA onset)[42]
- An approximately 25% increase of heart rate (beginning 1 second before RMMA onset), concomitant with
- An increase in EMG activity of the jaw opener muscle (eg, the suprahyoid muscle, probably responsible for mandible protrusion and airway opening), concomitant with
- An increase in the airflow amplitude visible as two big breaths preceding or concomitant with[58]

- An increase in diastolic and systolic blood pressure[59]
- An observable EMG incident in the jaw-closing muscles (masseter and temporalis), scored as RMMA with or without tooth-grinding sounds[4]; Almost 60% of RMMA episodes are followed in the 5 to 15 seconds after onset by swallowing (**Fig. 2**).[60]

Neurochemicals

Many neurochemicals and neurotransmitters may be involved in the genesis and modulation of jaw movements during sleep, especially those that participate in controlling motoneuron activity and regulating sleep and wake states (acetylcholine, noradrenalin, dopamine, orexin).[44,61] The dopaminergic system was first investigated after the early observation of tooth-grinding activity in a patient with Parkinson disease treated with L-dopa.[62] However, further studies using the dopamine precursor, L-dopa, and the dopaminergic agonist, bromocriptine, demonstrated only a modest effect of dopamine-related medications on SB.[63–65] Dopamine is not usually very active during sleep but it may be linked to sleep arousal reactivation.[66] Conversely, clonidine, an adrenergic agonist, reduced RMMA episodes by 60%, supporting the role of sympathetic-cardiac activation, adrenaline, and noradrenalin in SB genesis.[67] Because noradrenergic action is critical during non-REM sleep in the minutes preceding REM sleep onset, it may participate in the transition from non-REM to REM sleep, a state associated with muscle hypotonia.[68]

Other neurotransmitters, such as serotonin, gamma-aminobutyric acid, cholecystokinin, and orexin, may have a role in modulating RMMA during sleep. Ionic channels, receptors, and their cellular expression may also be involved in SB genesis. However,

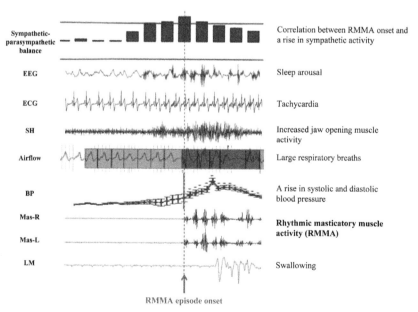

Fig. 2. Genesis of an RMMA episode. The cascade of physiologic events that precedes RMMA onset is shown (schematic representation). A detailed explanation is provided in the text. BP, blood pressure; ECG, electrocardiogram; LM, laryngeal movements; SH, EMG of the suprahyoid muscle; Mas-R and Mas-L, EMG of the right and left masseter muscles. (*Data from* Refs.[11,42,52,53,58,59])

either data are not yet available or the findings are supported by indirect evidence only, derived from case reports on drug and medication use. Prospective and randomized control experimental trials are needed before firm conclusions can be drawn on neurochemical participation in SB genesis.

Genetic Factors

There is little evidence for a genetic predisposition for SB. Children of patients with SB are more likely to be affected than children of individuals who never had SB or who suffer from wake-time bruxism only.[69] From 20% to 50% of patients with SB have a direct family member who ground his or her teeth in childhood, and childhood SB persists in adulthood in 87% of patients.[70,71] In a Finnish twin cohort study, higher concordance was found among monozygotic than dizygotic twins.[71,72]

Despite this early evidence of a genetic basis for SB, the inheritance pattern remains unknown, and no genetic marker has been identified to date. Further research on population-based samples is needed to explore and delineate the probable genetic component in SB genesis. It would be more likely related to genetic polymorphism than a single gene mechanism. Moreover, links to other wake and sleep behaviors would probably emerge.[73,74] It is worth noting that SB assessment tools in large populations, frequently based on a positive history of tooth grinding alone, have yet to be validated for acceptable sensitivity and specificity, especially in the general population. A clinical diagnosis of SB supported with portable systems or single-channel EMG recording is feasible and promising but still lacking in specificity.

Psychosocial Factors: Stress, Anxiety, and Behavior

Aside from a probable genetic predisposition, many other causal or risk factors may play a role in the genesis of SB activity. Psychosocial components in particular, such as anxiety and stress, have frequently been associated with SB.[29,75–79] Both child and adult patients reporting SB were found to have higher levels of urinary catecholamines (adrenaline, noradrenaline, dopamine) than controls.[80–82] These results were attributed to stress factors that activate the hypothalamic-adrenal axis, which controls the catecholamine release. Other studies, mainly questionnaire based, suggest that patients with SB may have maladaptive coping strategies: they seem to be more anxious, stressed, and task oriented as a result of their personality and coping style (eg, type A personality).[29,75,77,78,83,84] Especially in children, SB has been associated with behavioral habits and complaints. These complaints include neuroticism, perfectionism, aggressiveness, lack of concentration and attention (eg, at school), thought disorders, antisocial behaviors, and conduct disorders.[21,85–87] Moreover, all these psychosocial factors have been related to wake-time bruxism.[21] In fact, tooth clenching may be an adaptive or reactive learning behavior (to cope with stress, anxiety, and social life) that may also occur during sleep. However, the overlapping and interactions between wake-time and sleep-time bruxism are still matters of debate.

Alternatively, SB has been considered a tic, an automatism, a movement fragment, or tardive dyskinesia, which may manifest during wake time and persist during sleep.[88] In any case, the many and contrasting findings in the literature indicate that further research is needed to better understand the role of psychosocial factors in SB pathophysiology.[74,76]

Exogenous Factors and Comorbidities

Several exogenous factors and medical conditions have been associated with SB or bruxismlike activities during either sleep or wake time. The exogenous risk factors for

SB include alcohol consumption, cigarette smoking, caffeine intake, medication use (eg, selective serotonin reuptake inhibitor [SSRI]), and drug use (eg, ecstasy).[29,89–99] SB may also be observed in comorbidity with medical disorders, such as attention-deficit/hyperactivity disorder (ADHD)[100,101]; movement disorders (eg, Parkinson disease and Huntington disease)[102,103]; dementia[104–106]; epilepsy[107–109]; gastro-esophageal reflux[110]; and other sleep disorders, such as parasomnias (eg, sleep walking, sleep talking, enuresis, REM sleep behavior disorder [RBD]), periodic limb movements (PLM), RLS, and SDB (**Box 3**).[111–115] It remains to be assessed, however, whether these are cases of intersecting prevalence between 2 parallel disorders or if one condition causes or exacerbates the other.[116]

When SB is associated with medication or drug intake or with medical diseases, it is defined as secondary or iatrogenic SB. Conversely, in the absence of medical causes, SB is considered to be primary, or idiopathic, and it can in turn lead to several clinical consequences on the stomatognathic system, such as tooth wear, tooth damage, tooth fractures, muscle fatigue, orofacial pain, temporomandibular disorders (TMD), and headache.[4]

Box 3
SB and comorbidities

Parasomnias

    Enuresis

    Sleep talking

    Sleep walking

    RBD

Other sleep-related disorders

    Sleep-disordered breathing (snoring, obstructive sleep apnea)

    Sleep-related epilepsy

    PLM and RLS

    Sleep-related gastroesophageal reflux

Medical and psychological conditions

    Hypertrophic tonsils or adenoids

    Allergies

    ADHD

    Headaches

    Orofacial pain and temporomandibular disorders

    Stress and anxiety

    Neurologic and psychiatric disorders (eg, dementia, depression)

    Movement disorders (eg, Parkinson disease, oromandibular dystonia, tics)

Oral habits and parafunctions

    Tics

    Nail biting, pen biting, and so forth

    Wake-time tooth clenching

Data from Refs.[23,100–102,107,108,110,115,117–120]

SB, Orofacial Pain, and TMD

Orofacial pain is reported by from 66% to 84% of patients with SB.[117,118] However, the presence or intensity of pain does not seem to be directly correlated with the frequency of RMMA episodes.[23,119,121] In fact, patients with SB with a low frequency of RMMA (2–4 episodes per hour of sleep) seem to have higher risks for orofacial pain and headache than patients with SB with a high frequency of RMMA (>4 episodes per hour of sleep).[23,122] Furthermore, note that SB may coexist with wake-time tooth clenching and other oral parafunctions (eg, lip, cheek, or nail biting), which can also cause or contribute to the development and persistence of orofacial pain.[123–128]

SB has been largely considered a sign or cause of TMD in both adult and pediatric populations.[129–134] Several studies suggest that SB may play a role in TMD genesis, especially the myogenous component, because of muscle hyperactivity during sleep. Nevertheless, TMD pain and morning jaw-muscle pain may be different entities. Most patients with TMD report a pain intensity peak in the late afternoon, whereas patients with SB report transient masseter and temporalis muscle pain or soreness mainly in the morning.[23,135,136]

SB and Headaches

SB has been frequently associated with headaches.[21,113,120,137–141] In a questionnaire-based study, children with SB reported approximately 3 times more headaches than control subjects, with an odds ratio of 4.3.[21] From 30% to 50% of adult patients with SB complain of headache either in the morning (most frequently) or during the day.[138] However, the exact mechanism underlying the possible interactions between SB and headaches remains unknown. It can be hypothesized that SB, which is characterized by repetitive rhythmic and sustained contractions of the masticatory muscles during sleep, may cause tension-type headaches during the daytime. In fact, this comorbidity is controversial because of the overlap with forms of TMD pain and TMD-related headaches.[142,143] Furthermore, the presence of an underlying sleep disorder, such as SDB, has often been associated with both SB and headache. In this latter case, the role of intermittent hypoxia and hypercapnia and sleep fragmentation (after obstructive respiratory events) may be the actual cause of the headaches (**Fig. 3**). Alternatively, SB, headache, and SDB may share common risk factors or pathophysiological substrates without a specific cause-and-effect relationship. For example, it has been shown that children with headaches frequently have concomitant sleep problems, such as SB and SDB, and a higher incidence of TMD.[144,145]

SB and SDB

Although SB and SDB (eg, upper airway resistance, obstructive sleep apnea [OSA], and central sleep apnea) have frequently been associated, the possible cause-and-effect relationship has not yet been elucidated.[29,146–148] Two open clinical studies and one case report have provided indirect evidence for this relationship by showing

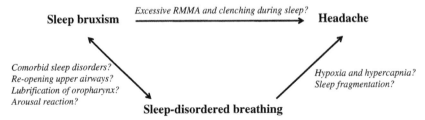

Fig. 3. Comorbid SB, headache, and SDB: putative mechanisms.

a decrease in SB after different SDB treatments (eg, adenotonsillectomy and continuous positive airway pressure).[149–151] These findings support the hypothesis that RMMA may be an oromotor activity that helps reinstate airway patency following an obstructive respiratory event during sleep.[58] An alternative hypothesis considers RMMA a physiologic motor event that is required to lubricate the oropharyngeal structures during sleep, a period when salivary flow and swallowing rate are normally reduced.[60,152] The factors that induce RMMA to reach abnormal frequency in patients with SB remain to be elucidated.

MANAGEMENT OF SB

No therapy to date has been proven effective to cure SB. The available treatment approaches aim at managing and preventing the harmful consequences of SB to the orofacial structures (**Table 3**).[153]

Behavioral Strategies

SB can be managed by behavioral strategies, including the avoidance of SB risk factors and triggers (eg, consumption of tobacco, alcohol, caffeine, and drugs), patient education (eg, control of wake-time oral parafunctions), relaxation techniques, sleep hygiene, hypnotherapy, biofeedback, and cognitive behavioral therapy.[154–158] However, most of these strategies have not been adequately tested in controlled trials. Nevertheless, a recent study showed that a new biofeedback device that applies electrical pulses to inhibit EMG activity in the temporalis muscle was effective in the short term in reducing EMG activity during sleep, without disrupting sleep quality.[155] In addition, a 12-week cognitive behavioral therapy session with patients with SB was found to reduce SB but showed no significant benefits over occlusal splint therapy.[156] Although these behavioral techniques have not yet shown clear or persistent effects, they seem to improve patients' well being and should be considered the first-line management approach in patients with SB.

Oral Appliances

To protect dental surfaces and relax the masticatory muscles, occlusal splints, either on the maxillary or the mandibular arch, have been extensively used in clinical practice. However, the exact mechanism of action is still under debate and there is no evidence to support their role in halting SB. Moreover, the lack of well-designed randomized controlled clinical trials and long-term studies in the literature makes it difficult to assess their effectiveness.[159] Most studies show a decrease (40%–50%) in the RMMA index in the first period of treatment (2–6 weeks), regardless of the type of occlusal splint.[24,160–162] However, the effect seems to be transitory, with values returning to baseline after a short time and the outcomes are highly variable between patients. Moreover, it has been reported that approximately 20% of patients with SB show increased EMG activity during sleep when wearing an occlusal splint, especially the soft mouth guard type.[163]

Occlusal and anterior tooth appliances (eg, the nociceptive trigeminal inhibition system, NTI [http://www.nti-tss.com]) are also used in cases of SB comorbid with orofacial pain and TMD to relief muscle and joint pain.[164–168] Their effectiveness is still controversial because they rarely halt RMMA occurrence.[169] However, it has been hypothesized that these devices may make patients more conscious of their oral parafunctional habits by altering proprioceptive inputs, thus, helping them reduce clenching activity, albeit mainly during wake time.[170,171] Patients with TMD seem to find relief with occlusal splints compared with other or no treatment, especially the most severe

Table 3
Management of SB

Clinical Approach	Functions	Potential Side Effects
Behavioral strategies		
• Patient education, sleep hygiene, relaxation techniques, hypnotherapy, biofeedback, and cognitive behavioral therapy	• Avoid SB risk factors (eg, smoking, alcohol, caffeine, drugs) • Control wake-time oral parafunctions • Improve sleep habits and sleep environment • Control and reduce stress and anxiety (coping) • Relax muscles and reduce EMG activity during sleep	• None identified to date
Intraoral appliances		
• Occlusal or stabilization splint • NTI	• Protect tooth surfaces • Reduce EMG activity (?)	• Impaired occlusion[a] • Increased SB activity • Posterior dental overeruption or anterior dental intrusion (for NTI)[a]
• Mandibular advancement appliances (commonly used for snoring and mild to moderate OSA)	• Reposition and stabilize the lower jaw, tongue, and soft tissues • Open the upper airway space	• Excessive salivation or dry mouth • Tenderness in the teeth, TMJ, muscles • Perception of abnormal occlusion in the morning • Occlusal changes (eg, reduced overjet and overbite)[a]
Pharmacotherapy (recommended in the short term only)		
	• Reduce SB activity + extra effects related to the kind of medication used (eg, hypnotic, analgesic)	Depends on the medication used: • Clonazepam: tolerance, physiologic dependence, fatigue, somnolence • Clonidine: hypotension • Botulinum toxin: risk of retrograde transportation from the site of injection to CNS with systemic side effects

Abbreviations: CNS, central nervous system; NTI, nociceptive trigeminal inhibition system; TMJ, temporomandibular joint.

[a] Only in long-term treatment.

Data from Lavigne G, Manzini C, Huynh NT. Sleep Bruxism. In: Kryger MH, Roth T, Dement WC, editors. Principles and practice of sleep medicine. 5th edition. St Louis (MO): Elsevier Saunders; 2011. p. 1129–39.

cases with TMD pain.[172] Physiotherapy sessions targeting the masticatory muscles may also be useful in cases of SB associated with orofacial pain or TMD.[173,174]

It is worth mentioning that occlusal appliances and anterior tooth splints are not free of unwanted side effects, including changes in dental occlusion, single tooth positioning, dental hypersensitiveness, and worsening of orofacial pain and SDB.[175] For example, in a pilot study of 10 patients with OSA, a maxillary occlusal splint was found to increase the hypopnea/apnea index in half of the patients, probably by reducing the intraoral space for the tongue, which changes the tongue position during sleep.[175] When SB is concomitant with OSA, or when SDB are suspected, a mandibular occlusal splint (custom made for the lower jaw) or a mandibular advancement appliance (MAA) would be preferable.

MAAs, which are currently used to treat snoring and mild to moderate forms of OSA, have also been tested in the short term to challenge the role of the airways in the genesis of RMMA episodes and to assess therapeutic benefits in patients with SB. An MAA was demonstrated effective in decreasing SB (up to 70%), especially when worn in advanced positions (50%–75% of the maximal protrusion).[176,177] They also seem to relieve daily morning headaches in patients with a low frequency of RMMA during sleep.[178] Although the use of an MAA for SB showed good effectiveness,[153] all these studies assessed the effect after short-term treatment only (2 weeks average). It remains to assess their effectiveness and side effects in long-term studies.[179,180]

Pharmacotherapy

Several medications and drugs have been associated with decreased or increased SB activity, supporting the probability of central mechanisms for SB genesis (**Box 4**).[89] In particular, the dopaminergic, serotoninergic, and adrenergic systems are thought to be involved in this orofacial motor activity. However, evidence is lacking on both the effectiveness and safety of using medications in patients with SB. Therefore, in symptomatic and most severe patients, pharmacologic treatments should be considered as a short-term therapy only.[4]

A recent placebo-controlled study demonstrated a 40% reduction in SB activity with an acute dose of clonazepam (1 mg).[181,182] Clonazepam is a benzodiazepine with hypnotic, anxiolytic, anticonvulsive, and myorelaxant effects. It acts at various levels of the central nervous system. The beneficial effect on SB genesis may result from actions on different systems linked to muscle activity, emotions, and behaviors. However, there are no available data on long-term treatment or potential side effects, such as sleepiness (risk of transportation or work-related accidents), pharmacobehavioral tolerance, and dependence.

Antidepressant drugs have also been recommended for SB as well as for chronic orofacial pain. However, there is little evidence to support their use. Low doses of amitriptyline (a tricyclic antidepressant) were found to be ineffective against SB,[189,190] and SSRI medications (eg, fluoxetine, sertraline, paroxetine) actually increased tooth grinding and clenching.[95,183,191]

Adrenergic beta-blockers, such as propranolol, were shown to be ineffective on SB.[67] Conversely, an acute dose (0.3 mg) of the alpha$_2$-adrenergic agonist, clonidine, reduced SB by 60%, supporting the role of autonomic cardiac activation in the genesis of this sleep-related motor disorder. However, clonidine is associated with sleep structure changes (eg, less REM sleep) and severe morning hypotension.[56,67] Its use for SB therapy is highly controversial.

Anecdotal reports suggest a positive effect on SB of gabapentin,[184] tiagabine,[192] buspirone,[193] topiramate,[185] and botulinum toxin.[186,187] However, their effectiveness and safety need to be assessed in randomized controlled clinical trials. Potential candidates for more specific or more potent medications are substances that regulate the wake-sleep balance (eg, acetylcholine, noradrenaline, dopamine, orexin, histamine, serotonin), ionic channels, and cellular receptors (on neurons and glia).

> **Box 4**
> **Effect of medications and chemical substances on SB or SB-like activity[a]**
>
> *Increased SB activity*
> - SSRI (eg, paroxetine, fluoxetine, sertraline)
> - Norepinephrine-selective reuptake inhibitors (eg, venlafaxine)
> - Antipsychotic (eg, haloperidol)
> - Flunarizine
> - Amphetamines (eg, methylphenidate)
> - 3,4-methylenedioxymethamphetamine (ecstasy)
> - Cocaine
> - Caffeine
> - Nicotine
> - Alcohol
>
> *Decreased SB activity*
> - Clonazepam
> - Diazepam
> - Methocarbamol
> - Buspirone
> - Levodopa
> - Pergolide
> - Clonidine
> - Gabapentin
> - Topiramate
> - Botulinum toxin
>
> *No effect on SB activity*
> - Propranolol, bromocriptine, L-tryptophan
>
> [a] The scientific evidence is based primarily on case reports (except for 2 randomized controlled clinical trials with PSG [Huynh 2006; Saletu 2010]). No long-term studies have assessed safety or benefits.
>   *Data from* Refs.[64,67,89–91,97,181–188]

SUMMARY

SB is a common sleep-related disorder that can be highly distressing because of several harmful consequences to the stomatognathic system, including tooth damage, headaches, muscle pain, and TMD. Dental clinicians are responsible for detecting and preventing these detrimental consequences to patients' oral health. However, SB is much more than tooth wear. Patients with SB need to be screened for other comorbid medical conditions (eg, SDB, insomnia, ADHD, depression, mood disorders, gastroesophageal reflux) before undertaking any treatment approach, especially pharmacotherapy. Because underlying disorders and medication intake may interfere with motor activities during sleep, they need to be assessed before other treatments are recommended. Furthermore, if a medical comorbidity is

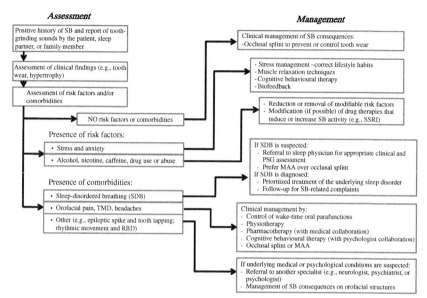

Assessment   *Management*

Fig. 4. Algorithm for the clinical assessment and management of SB.

diagnosed (eg, SDB), the therapeutic approach should primarily address the medical disorder while managing the consequences of SB (**Fig. 4**).

CASE STUDY
History and Clinical Examination

A 43-year-old woman complains about tooth grinding during sleep almost nightly. The patient has normal weight and no medical or neurologic diseases but smokes approximately 20 cigarettes a day. She judges herself as highly stressed at work. She reports occasional transient morning jaw-muscle pain, a sensation of jaw locking, and uncomfortable dental occlusion on awakening. However, these symptoms tend to disappear after 30 to 60 minutes and they do not particularly disturb the patient's quality of life. The patient reports good quality of sleep, but tooth-grinding noises and moderate snoring disturb her husband's sleep. The patient's chief complaint is the severe tooth damage she has observed on her dental surfaces, with a negative impact on her esthetic profile, to the point that she does not feel like smiling anymore.

Assessment and Diagnosis

At the clinical examination, severe tooth wear, masseter muscle hypertrophy, and mild pain on palpation at the lateral pterygoid muscles are observed. The patient presents a dental and skeletal class II, a narrow and deep palate, and a Mallampati score of III. The Epworth Sleepiness Scale score indicates a low likelihood of daytime sleepiness, and no other SDB-related signs or symptoms are charted. Based on the patient's and her husband's reports of tooth-grinding sounds and the presence of relevant signs and symptoms, the patient is clinically diagnosed with SB and anatomic predisposition for SDB (history of snoring, retrognathia, and narrow and deep palate, Mallampati III). A PSG evaluation is not mandatory at the moment because the patient does not present any SDB-related symptoms (except for snoring). However, a long-term follow-up is recommended because the risk of SDB increases in women after menopause.

Suggested Clinical Management

The patient should be informed on the characteristics and consequences of SB as well as the available management options. First, cigarette smoking and other possible triggers should be avoided or reduced. Behavioral strategies should be tried to decrease stress, improve coping strategies, and relax the masticatory muscles. To control and prevent tooth wear, an intraoral appliance is recommended. However, because the patient is already a snorer and presents anatomic risk factors for SDB, an MAA would be preferable to an occlusal or stabilization splint. To address esthetic concerns, conservative and prosthodontic treatments should be planned. Follow-up visits must be scheduled to customize and adjust the MAA, verify the patient's general and oral status (stress level), and prevent SB consequences (tooth wear, pain) from worsening.

REFERENCES

1. The glossary of prosthodontic terms. J Prosthet Dent 2005;94(1):10–92.
2. De Leeuw R. Orofacial pain. Guidelines for assessment, diagnosis and management. 4th edition. Chicago: Quintessence; 2008.
3. American Academy of Sleep Medicine (AASM), editor. International classification of sleep disorders. Diagnosis and coding manual. (ICSD-2). Section on sleep related bruxism. 2nd edition. Westchester(IL): American Academy of Sleep Medicine; 2005. p. 189–92.
4. Lavigne G, Manzini C, Huynh NT. Sleep bruxism. In: Kryger MH, Roth T, Dement WC, editors. Principles and practice of sleep medicine. 5th edition. St Louis (MO): Elsevier Saunders; 2011. p. 1129–39.
5. Lavigne GJ, Rompre PH, Poirier G, et al. Rhythmic masticatory muscle activity during sleep in humans. J Dent Res 2001;80(2):443–8.
6. De Laat A, Macaluso GM. Sleep bruxism as a motor disorder. Mov Disord 2002; 17(Suppl 2):S67–9.
7. Kato T, Thie NM, Montplaisir JY, et al. Bruxism and orofacial movements during sleep. Dent Clin North Am 2001;45(4):657–84.
8. Dutra KM, Pereira FJ Jr, Rompre PH, et al. Oro-facial activities in sleep bruxism patients and in normal subjects: a controlled polygraphic and audio-video study. J Oral Rehabil 2009;36(2):86–92.
9. Lavigne GJ, Rompre PH, Montplaisir JY. Sleep bruxism: validity of clinical research diagnostic criteria in a controlled polysomnographic study. J Dent Res 1996;75(1):546–52.
10. Walters AS, Lavigne G, Hening W, et al. The scoring of movements in sleep. J Clin Sleep Med 2007;3(2):155–67.
11. Kato T, Rompre P, Montplaisir JY, et al. Sleep bruxism: an oromotor activity secondary to micro-arousal. J Dent Res 2001;80(10):1940–4.
12. Carra MC, Rompre PH, Kato T, et al. Sleep bruxism and sleep arousal: an experimental challenge to assess the role of cyclic alternating pattern. J Oral Rehabil 2011;38(9):635–42.
13. Iber C, Anacoli-Israel S, Chesson A, et al. The AASM manual for the scoring of sleep and associated events: rules, terminology and technical specifications. Westchester (IL): American Academy of Sleep Medicine (AASM); 2007.
14. Koyano K, Tsukiyama Y, Ichiki R, et al. Assessment of bruxism in the clinic. J Oral Rehabil 2008;35(7):495–508.
15. Lavigne GJ, Khoury S, Abe S, et al. Bruxism physiology and pathology: an overview for clinicians. J Oral Rehabil 2008;35(7):476–94.

16. Abe S, Yamaguchi T, Rompre PH, et al. Tooth wear in young subjects: a discriminator between sleep bruxers and controls? Int J Prosthodont 2009;22(4): 342–50.

17. Johansson A, Johansson AK, Omar R, et al. Rehabilitation of the worn dentition. J Oral Rehabil 2008;35(7):548–66.

18. Pergamalian A, Rudy TE, Zaki HS, et al. The association between wear facets, bruxism, and severity of facial pain in patients with temporomandibular disorders. J Prosthet Dent 2003;90(2):194–200.

19. Chan AS, Lee RW, Cistulli PA. Sleep-related breathing disorders. In: Lavigne GJ, Cistulli PA, Smith MT, editors. Sleep medicine for dentists. A practical overview. Hanover Park (IL): Quintessence Publishing Co, Inc; 2009. p. 35–40.

20. Philip P, Gross CE, Taillard J, et al. An animal model of a spontaneously reversible obstructive sleep apnea syndrome in the monkey. Neurobiol Dis 2005;20(2): 428–31.

21. Carra MC, Huynh N, Morton P, et al. Prevalence and risk factors of sleep bruxism and wake-time tooth clenching in a 7- to 17-yr-old population. Eur J Oral Sci 2011;119(5):386–94.

22. Hirshkowitz M, Kryger MH. Monitoring techniques for evaluating suspected sleep-disordered breathing. In: Kryger MH, Roth T, Dement WC, editors. Principles and practice of sleep medicine. 5th edition. St Louis (MO): Elsevier Saunders; 2011. p. 1610–23.

23. Rompre PH, Daigle-Landry D, Guitard F, et al. Identification of a sleep bruxism subgroup with a higher risk of pain. J Dent Res 2007;86(9):837–42.

24. van der Zaag J, Lobbezoo F, Wicks DJ, et al. Controlled assessment of the efficacy of occlusal stabilization splints on sleep bruxism. J Orofac Pain 2005; 19(2):151–8.

25. Ikeda T, Nishigawa K, Kondo K, et al. Criteria for the detection of sleep-associated bruxism in humans. J Orofac Pain 1996;10(3):270–82.

26. Gallo LM, Lavigne G, Rompre P, et al. Reliability of scoring EMG orofacial events: polysomnography compared with ambulatory recordings. J Sleep Res 1997;6(4):259–63.

27. Koyano K, Tsukiyama Y. Clinical approach to diagnosis of sleep bruxism. In: Lavigne GJ, Cistulli PA, Smith MT, editors. Sleep medicine for dentists. A practical overview. 1st edition. Hanover Park (IL): Quintessence Publishing Co, Inc; 2009. p. 109–16.

28. Lavigne GJ, Montplaisir JY. Restless legs syndrome and sleep bruxism: prevalence and association among Canadians. Sleep 1994;17(8):739–43.

29. Ohayon MM, Li KK, Guilleminault C. Risk factors for sleep bruxism in the general population. Chest 2001;119(1):53–61.

30. Simola P, Niskakangas M, Liukkonen K, et al. Sleep problems and daytime tiredness in Finnish preschool-aged children-a community survey. Child Care Health Dev 2010;36(6):805–11.

31. Castelo PM, Barbosa TS, Gaviao MB. Quality of life evaluation of children with sleep bruxism. BMC Oral Health 2010;10:16.

32. Strausz T, Ahlberg J, Lobbezoo F, et al. Awareness of tooth grinding and clenching from adolescence to young adulthood: a nine-year follow-up. J Oral Rehabil 2010;37(7):497–500.

33. Serra-Negra JM, Paiva SM, Seabra AP, et al. Prevalence of sleep bruxism in a group of Brazilian school children. Eur Arch Paediatr Dent 2010;11(4):192–5.

34. Laberge L, Tremblay RE, Vitaro F, et al. Development of parasomnias from childhood to early adolescence. Pediatrics 2000;106(1 Pt 1):67–74.

35. Petit D, Touchette E, Tremblay RE, et al. Dyssomnias and parasomnias in early childhood. Pediatrics 2007;119(5):e1016–25.
36. Cheifetz AT, Osganian SK, Allred EN, et al. Prevalence of bruxism and associated correlates in children as reported by parents. J Dent Child (Chic) 2005; 72(2):67–73.
37. Ng DK, Kwok KL, Cheung JM, et al. Prevalence of sleep problems in Hong Kong primary school children: a community-based telephone survey. Chest 2005; 128(3):1315–23.
38. Carlsson GE, Egermark I, Magnusson T. Predictors of bruxism, other oral parafunctions, and tooth wear over a 20-year follow-up period. J Orofac Pain 2003; 17(1):50–7.
39. Agerberg G, Bergenholtz A. Craniomandibular disorders in adult populations of West Bothnia, Sweden. Acta Odontol Scand 1989;47(3):129–40.
40. Mobilio N, Casetta I, Cesnik E, et al. Prevalence of self-reported symptoms related to temporomandibular disorders in an Italian population. J Oral Rehabil 2011;38(12):884–90.
41. Glaros AG. Incidence of diurnal and nocturnal bruxism. J Prosthet Dent 1981; 45(5):545–9.
42. Lavigne GJ, Huynh N, Kato T, et al. Genesis of sleep bruxism: motor and autonomic-cardiac interactions. Arch Oral Biol 2007;52(4):381–4.
43. Gastaldo E, Quatrale R, Graziani A, et al. The excitability of the trigeminal motor system in sleep bruxism: a transcranial magnetic stimulation and brainstem reflex study. J Orofac Pain 2006;20(2):145–55.
44. Lavigne GJ, Kato T, Kolta A, et al. Neurobiological mechanisms involved in sleep bruxism. Crit Rev Oral Biol Med 2003;14(1):30–46.
45. Kato T, Thie NM, Huynh N, et al. Topical review: sleep bruxism and the role of peripheral sensory influences. J Orofac Pain 2003;17(3):191–213.
46. Lobbezoo F, Naeije M. Bruxism is mainly regulated centrally, not peripherally. J Oral Rehabil 2001;28(12):1085–91.
47. Lavigne G, Toumilehto H, Macaluso GM. Pathophysiology of sleep bruxism. In: Lavigne GJ, Cistulli PA, Smith MT, editors. Sleep medicine for dentists. A practical overview. Hanover Park (IL): Quintessence Publishing Co, Inc; 2009. p. 117–24.
48. Macaluso GM, Guerra P, Di Giovanni G, et al. Sleep bruxism is a disorder related to periodic arousals during sleep. J Dent Res 1998;77(4):565–73.
49. Reding GR, Zepelin H, Robinson JE Jr, et al. Nocturnal teeth-grinding: all-night psychophysiologic studies. J Dent Res 1968;47(5):786–97.
50. Satoh T, Harada Y. Tooth-grinding during sleep as an arousal reaction. Experientia 1971;27(7):785–6.
51. Satoh T, Harada Y. Electrophysiological study on tooth-grinding during sleep. Electroencephalogr Clin Neurophysiol 1973;35(3):267–75.
52. Huynh N, Kato T, Rompre PH, et al. Sleep bruxism is associated to micro-arousals and an increase in cardiac sympathetic activity. J Sleep Res 2006; 15(3):339–46.
53. Kato T, Montplaisir JY, Guitard F, et al. Evidence that experimentally induced sleep bruxism is a consequence of transient arousal. J Dent Res 2003;82(4): 284–8.
54. Terzano MG, Parrino L. Origin and significance of the cyclic alternating pattern (CAP). Review article. Sleep Med Rev 2000;4(1):101–23.
55. Parrino L, Ferri R, Bruni O, et al. Cyclic alternating pattern (CAP): the marker of sleep instability. Sleep Med Rev 2012;16(1):27–45.

56. Carra MC, Macaluso GM, Rompre PH, et al. Clonidine has a paradoxical effect on cyclic arousal and sleep bruxism during NREM sleep. Sleep 2010;33(12):1711–6.
57. Marthol H, Reich S, Jacke J, et al. Enhanced sympathetic cardiac modulation in bruxism patients. Clin Auton Res 2006;16(4):276–80.
58. Khoury S, Rouleau GA, Rompre PH, et al. A significant increase in breathing amplitude precedes sleep bruxism. Chest 2008;134(2):332–7.
59. Nashed A, Lanfranchi P, Rompré P, et al. Sleep bruxism is associated with a rise in arterial blood pressure. Sleep 2012;35(4), in press.
60. Miyawaki S, Lavigne GJ, Pierre M, et al. Association between sleep bruxism, swallowing-related laryngeal movement, and sleep positions. Sleep 2003; 26(4):461–5.
61. Saper CB, Scammell TE, Lu J. Hypothalamic regulation of sleep and circadian rhythms. Nature 2005;437(7063):1257–63.
62. Magee KR. Bruxism related to levodopa therapy. JAMA 1970;214(1):147.
63. Lavigne GJ, Soucy JP, Lobbezoo F, et al. Double-blind, crossover, placebo-controlled trial of bromocriptine in patients with sleep bruxism. Clin Neurophar-macol 2001;24(3):145–9.
64. Lobbezoo F, Lavigne GJ, Tanguay R, et al. The effect of catecholamine precursor L-dopa on sleep bruxism: a controlled clinical trial. Mov Disord 1997;12(1):73–8.
65. Lobbezoo F, Soucy JP, Montplaisir JY, et al. Striatal D2 receptor binding in sleep bruxism: a controlled study with iodine-123-iodobenzamide and single-photon-emission computed tomography. J Dent Res 1996;75(10):1804–10.
66. McCarley RW. Neurobiology of REM and NREM sleep. Sleep Med 2007;8(4): 302–30.
67. Huynh N, Lavigne GJ, Lanfranchi PA, et al. The effect of 2 sympatholytic medi-cations–propranolol and clonidine–on sleep bruxism: experimental randomized controlled studies. Sleep 2006;29(3):307–16.
68. Pal D, Mallick BN. Neural mechanism of rapid eye movement sleep generation with reference to REM-OFF neurons in locus coeruleus. Indian J Med Res 2007; 125(6):721–39.
69. Reding GR, Rubright WC, Zimmerman SO. Incidence of bruxism. J Dent Res 1966;45(4):1198–204.
70. Lindqvist B. Bruxism in twins. Acta Odontol Scand 1974;32(3):177–87.
71. Hublin C, Kaprio J, Partinen M, et al. Sleep bruxism based on self-report in a nationwide twin cohort. J Sleep Res 1998;7(1):61–7.
72. Hublin C, Kaprio J. Genetic aspects and genetic epidemiology of parasomnias. Sleep Med Rev 2003;7(5):413–21.
73. Faraco J, Mignot E. Genetics of sleep and sleep disorders in humans. In: Kryger MH, Roth T, Dement WC, editors. Principles and practice of sleep medi-cine. 5th edition. St Louis (MO): Elsevier Saunders; 2011. p. 184–98.
74. Landolt H, Dijk DJ. Genetic basis of sleep in healthy humans. In: Kryger MH, Roth T, Dement WC, editors. Principles and practice of sleep medicine. 5th edition. St Louis (MO): Elsevier Saunders; 2011. p. 175–83.
75. Winocur E, Uziel N, Lisha T, et al. Self-reported bruxism - associations with perceived stress, motivation for control, dental anxiety and gagging. J Oral Re-habil 2011;38(1):3–11.
76. Manfredini D, Lobbezoo F. Role of psychosocial factors in the etiology of bruxism. J Orofac Pain 2009;23(2):153–66.
77. Pingitore G, Chrobak V, Petrie J. The social and psychologic factors of bruxism. J Prosthet Dent 1991;65(3):443–6.

78. Schneider C, Schaefer R, Ommerborn MA, et al. Maladaptive coping strategies in patients with bruxism compared to non-bruxing controls. Int J Behav Med 2007;14(4):257–61.

79. Sato C, Sato S, Takashina H, et al. Bruxism affects stress responses in stressed rats. Clin Oral Investig 2010;14(2):153–60.

80. Seraidarian P, Seraidarian PI, das Neves Cavalcanti B, et al. Urinary levels of catecholamines among individuals with and without sleep bruxism. Sleep Breath 2009;13(1):85–8.

81. Vanderas AP, Menenakou M, Kouimtzis T, et al. Urinary catecholamine levels and bruxism in children. J Oral Rehabil 1999;26(2):103–10.

82. Clark GT, Rugh JD, Handelman SL. Nocturnal masseter muscle activity and urinary catecholamine levels in bruxers. J Dent Res 1980;59(10):1571–6.

83. Major M, Rompre PH, Guitard F, et al. A controlled daytime challenge of motor performance and vigilance in sleep bruxers. J Dent Res 1999;78(11):1754–62.

84. Giraki M, Schneider C, Schafer R, et al. Correlation between stress, stress-coping and current sleep bruxism. Head Face Med 2010;6:2.

85. Katayoun E, Sima F, Naser V, et al. Study of the relationship of psychosocial disorders to bruxism in adolescents. J Indian Soc Pedod Prev Dent 2008;26(Suppl 3):S91–7.

86. Restrepo CC, Vasquez LM, Alvarez M, et al. Personality traits and temporomandibular disorders in a group of children with bruxing behaviour. J Oral Rehabil 2008;35(8):585–93.

87. Serra-Negra JM, Ramos-Jorge ML, Flores-Mendoza CE, et al. Influence of psychosocial factors on the development of sleep bruxism among children. Int J Paediatr Dent 2009;19(5):309–17.

88. Adams RD, Victor M. Principle of neurology. 5th edition. New York: McGraw-Hill, Inc; 1993. p. 348.

89. Winocur E, Gavish A, Voikovitch M, et al. Drugs and bruxism: a critical review. J Orofac Pain 2003;17(2):99–111.

90. Winocur E, Gavish A, Volfin G, et al. Oral motor parafunctions among heavy drug addicts and their effects on signs and symptoms of temporomandibular disorders. J Orofac Pain 2001;15(1):56–63.

91. Dinis-Oliveira RJ, Caldas I, Carvalho F, et al. Bruxism after 3,4-methylene-dioxymethamphetamine (ecstasy) abuse. Clin Toxicol (Phila) 2010;48(8):863–4.

92. Sabuncuoglu O, Ekinci O, Berkem M. Fluoxetine-induced sleep bruxism in an adolescent treated with buspirone: a case report. Spec Care Dentist 2009;29(5):215–7.

93. Gerber PE, Lynd LD. Selective serotonin-reuptake inhibitor-induced movement disorders. Ann Pharmacother 1998;32(6):692–8.

94. Romanelli F, Adler DA, Bungay KM. Possible paroxetine-induced bruxism. Ann Pharmacother 1996;30(11):1246–8.

95. Ellison JM, Stanziani P. SSRI-associated nocturnal bruxism in four patients. J Clin Psychiatry 1993;54(11):432–4.

96. Lavigne GL, Lobbezoo F, Rompre PH, et al. Cigarette smoking as a risk factor or an exacerbating factor for restless legs syndrome and sleep bruxism. Sleep 1997;20(4):290–3.

97. Amir I, Hermesh H, Gavish A. Bruxism secondary to antipsychotic drug exposure: a positive response to propranolol. Clin Neuropharmacol 1997;20(1):86–9.

98. Rintakoski K, Ahlberg J, Hublin C, et al. Bruxism is associated with nicotine dependence: a nationwide Finnish twin cohort study. Nicotine Tob Res 2010; 12(12):1254–60.

99. Madrid G, Madrid S, Vranesh JG, et al. Cigarette smoking and bruxism. Percept Mot Skills 1998;87(3 Pt 1):898.

100. Silvestri R, Gagliano A, Arico I, et al. Sleep disorders in children with attention-deficit/hyperactivity disorder (ADHD) recorded overnight by video-polysomnography. Sleep Med 2009;10(10):1132–8.

101. Herrera M, Valencia I, Grant M, et al. Bruxism in children: effect on sleep architecture and daytime cognitive performance and behavior. Sleep 2006;29(9): 1143–8.

102. Tan EK, Jankovic J, Ondo W. Bruxism in Huntington's disease. Mov Disord 2000; 15(1):171–3.

103. Srivastava T, Ahuja M, Srivastava M, et al. Bruxism as presenting feature of Parkinson's disease. J Assoc Physicians India 2002;50:457.

104. Kwak YT, Han IW, Lee PH, et al. Associated conditions and clinical significance of awake bruxism. Geriatr Gerontol Int 2009;9(4):382–90.

105. Stewart JT, Thomas JE, Williams LS. Severe bruxism in a demented patient. South Med J 1993;86(4):476–7.

106. Trevathan E, Naidu S. The clinical recognition and differential diagnosis of Rett syndrome. J Child Neurol 1988;3(Suppl):S6–16.

107. Meletti S, Cantalupo G, Volpi L, et al. Rhythmic teeth grinding induced by temporal lobe seizures. Neurology 2004;62(12):2306–9.

108. Bisulli F, Vignatelli L, Naldi I, et al. Increased frequency of arousal parasomnias in families with nocturnal frontal lobe epilepsy: a common mechanism? Epilepsia 2010;51(9):1852–60.

109. Tinuper P, Provini F, Bisulli F, et al. Movement disorders in sleep: guidelines for differentiating epileptic from non-epileptic motor phenomena arising from sleep. Sleep Med Rev 2007;11(4):255–67.

110. Miyawaki S, Tanimoto Y, Araki Y, et al. Association between nocturnal bruxism and gastroesophageal reflux. Sleep 2003;26(7):888–92.

111. Lucchesi LM, Speciali JG, Santos-Silva R, et al. Nocturnal awakening with headache and its relationship with sleep disorders in a population-based sample of adult inhabitants of Sao Paulo City, Brazil. Cephalalgia 2010;30(12):1477–85.

112. Montplaisir J, Lapierre O, Lavigne G. The restless leg syndrome: a condition associated with periodic or aperiodic slowing of the EEG. Neurophysiol Clin 1994;24(2):131–40 [in French].

113. Miller VA, Palermo TM, Powers SW, et al. Migraine headaches and sleep disturbances in children. Headache 2003;43(4):362–8.

114. Sjoholm TT, Lowe AA, Miyamoto K, et al. Sleep bruxism in patients with sleep-disordered breathing. Arch Oral Biol 2000;45(10):889–96.

115. Sforza E, Zucconi M, Petronelli R, et al. REM sleep behavioral disorders. Eur Neurol 1988;28(5):295–300.

116. Reutens S, Sachdev PS. Periodic limb movements and other movement disorders in sleep: neuropsychiatric dimensions. Int Rev Psychiatry 2005;17(4): 283–92.

117. Bader G, Lavigne G. Sleep bruxism; an overview of an oromandibular sleep movement disorder. Review article. Sleep Med Rev 2000;4(1):27–43.

118. Camparis CM, Siqueira JT. Sleep bruxism: clinical aspects and characteristics in patients with and without chronic orofacial pain. Oral Surg Oral Med Oral Pathol Oral Radiol Endod 2006;101(2):188–93.

119. Rossetti LM, Pereira de Araujo Cdos R, Rossetti PH, et al. Association between rhythmic masticatory muscle activity during sleep and masticatory myofascial pain: a polysomnographic study. J Orofac Pain 2008;22(3):190–200.

120. Bruni O, Fabrizi P, Ottaviano S, et al. Prevalence of sleep disorders in childhood and adolescence with headache: a case-control study. Cephalalgia 1997;17(4): 492–8.

121. Nagamatsu-Sakaguchi C, Minakuchi H, Clark GT, et al. Relationship between the frequency of sleep bruxism and the prevalence of signs and symptoms of temporomandibular disorders in an adolescent population. Int J Prosthodont 2008;21(4):292–8.

122. Huynh N, Khoury S, Rompré PH, et al. Prevalence of headache and neck pain in a sleep bruxism population investigated in a sleep laboratory. Sleep 2006; 29(Abstract Suppl):A282.

123. Svensson P, Burgaard A, Schlosser S. Fatigue and pain in human jaw muscles during a sustained, low-intensity clenching task. Arch Oral Biol 2001;46(8):773–7.

124. Glaros AG, Burton E. Parafunctional clenching, pain, and effort in temporomandibular disorders. J Behav Med 2004;27(1):91–100.

125. McMillan AS, Lawson ET. Effect of tooth clenching and jaw opening on pain-pressure thresholds in the human jaw muscles. J Orofac Pain 1994;8(3):250–7.

126. Magnusson T, Egermark I, Carlsson GE. A longitudinal epidemiologic study of signs and symptoms of temporomandibular disorders from 15 to 35 years of age. J Orofac Pain 2000;14(4):310–9.

127. Velly AM, Gornitsky M, Philippe P. Contributing factors to chronic myofascial pain: a case-control study. Pain 2003;104(3):491–9.

128. Macfarlane TV, Kenealy P, Kingdon HA, et al. Orofacial pain in young adults and associated childhood and adulthood factors: results of the population study, Wales, United Kingdom. Community Dent Oral Epidemiol 2009;37(5):438–50.

129. Pereira LJ, Costa RC, Franca JP, et al. Risk indicators for signs and symptoms of temporomandibular dysfunction in children. J Clin Pediatr Dent 2009;34(1):81–6.

130. Pereira LJ, Pereira-Cenci T, Del Bel Cury AA, et al. Risk indicators of temporomandibular disorder incidences in early adolescence. Pediatr Dent 2010; 32(4):324–8.

131. Rugh JD, Harlan J. Nocturnal bruxism and temporomandibular disorders. Adv Neurol 1988;49:329–41.

132. Goulet JP, Clark GT, Flack VF, et al. The reproducibility of muscle and joint tenderness detection methods and maximum mandibular movement measurement for the temporomandibular system. J Orofac Pain 1998;12(1):17–26.

133. Barbosa Tde S, Miyakoda LS, Pocztaruk Rde L, et al. Temporomandibular disorders and bruxism in childhood and adolescence: review of the literature. Int J Pediatr Otorhinolaryngol 2008;72(3):299–314.

134. Miyake R, Ohkubo R, Takehara J, et al. Oral parafunctions and association with symptoms of temporomandibular disorders in Japanese university students. J Oral Rehabil 2004;31(6):518–23.

135. Dao TT, Lund JP, Lavigne GJ. Comparison of pain and quality of life in bruxers and patients with myofascial pain of the masticatory muscles. J Orofac Pain 1994;8(4):350–6.

136. Glaros AG, Williams K, Lausten L. Diurnal variation in pain reports in temporomandibular disorder patients and control subjects. J Orofac Pain 2008;22(2): 115–21.

137. Vendrame M, Kaleyias J, Valencia I, et al. Polysomnographic findings in children with headaches. Pediatr Neurol 2008;39(1):6–11.

138. Lavigne G, Palla S. Transient morning headache: recognizing the role of sleep bruxism and sleep-disordered breathing. J Am Dent Assoc 2010; 141(3):297–9.

139. Zarowski M, Mlodzikowska-Albrecht J, Steinborn B. The sleep habits and sleep disorders in children with headache. Adv Med Sci 2007;52(Suppl 1):194–6.

140. Biondi DM. Headaches and their relationship to sleep. Dent Clin North Am 2001; 45(4):685–700.

141. Bailey DR. Tension headache and bruxism in the sleep disordered patient. Cranio 1990;8(2):174–82.

142. Macfarlane TV, Gray RJ, Kincey J, et al. Factors associated with the temporomandibular disorder, pain dysfunction syndrome (PDS): Manchester case-control study. Oral Dis 2001;7(6):321–30.

143. Olesen J, Lipton RB. Headache classification update 2004. Curr Opin Neurol 2004;17:275–82.

144. Isik U, Ersu RH, Ay P, et al. Prevalence of headache and its association with sleep disorders in children. Pediatr Neurol 2007;36(3):146–51.

145. Liljestrom MR, Le Bell Y, Anttila P, et al. Headache children with temporomandibular disorders have several types of pain and other symptoms. Cephalalgia 2005;25(11):1054–60.

146. Sheldon SH. Obstructive sleep apnea and bruxism in children. Sleep Med Clin 2010;5(1):163–8.

147. Eitner S, Urschitz MS, Guenther A, et al. Sleep problems and daytime somnolence in a German population-based sample of snoring school-aged children. J Sleep Res 2007;16(1):96–101.

148. Grechi TH, Trawitzki LV, de Felicio CM, et al. Bruxism in children with nasal obstruction. Int J Pediatr Otorhinolaryngol 2008;72(3):391–6.

149. DiFrancesco RC, Junqueira PA, Trezza PM, et al. Improvement of bruxism after T & A surgery. Int J Pediatr Otorhinolaryngol 2004;68(4):441–5.

150. Eftekharian A, Raad N, Gholami-Ghasri N. Bruxism and adenotonsillectomy. Int J Pediatr Otorhinolaryngol 2008;72(4):509–11.

151. Oksenberg A, Arons E. Sleep bruxism related to obstructive sleep apnea: the effect of continuous positive airway pressure. Sleep Med 2002;3(6):513–5.

152. Thie NM, Kato T, Bader G, et al. The significance of saliva during sleep and the relevance of oromotor movements. Sleep Med Rev 2002;6(3):213–27.

153. Huynh N, Manzini C, Rompre PH, et al. Weighing the potential effectiveness of various treatments for sleep bruxism. J Can Dent Assoc 2007;73(8):727–30.

154. Shulman J. Teaching patients how to stop bruxing habits. J Am Dent Assoc 2001;132(9):1275–7.

155. Jadidi F, Castrillon E, Svensson P. Effect of conditioning electrical stimuli on temporalis electromyographic activity during sleep. J Oral Rehabil 2008;35(3): 171–83.

156. Ommerborn MA, Schneider C, Giraki M, et al. Effects of an occlusal splint compared with cognitive-behavioral treatment on sleep bruxism activity. Eur J Oral Sci 2007;115(1):7–14.

157. Wieselmann-Penkner K, Janda M, Lorenzoni M, et al. A comparison of the muscular relaxation effect of TENS and EMG-biofeedback in patients with bruxism. J Oral Rehabil 2001;28(9):849–53.

158. Lobbezoo F, van der Zaag J, van Selms MK, et al. Principles for the management of bruxism. J Oral Rehabil 2008;35(7):509–23.

159. Macedo CR, Silva AB, Machado MA, et al. Occlusal splints for treating sleep bruxism (tooth grinding). Cochrane Database Syst Rev 2007;4:CD005514.

160. Nascimento LL, Amorim CF, Giannasi LC, et al. Occlusal splint for sleep bruxism: an electromyographic associated to Helkimo index evaluation. Sleep Breath 2008;12(3):275–80.

161. Harada T, Ichiki R, Tsukiyama Y, et al. The effect of oral splint devices on sleep bruxism: a 6-week observation with an ambulatory electromyographic recording device. J Oral Rehabil 2006;33(7):482–8.

162. Dube C, Rompre PH, Manzini C, et al. Quantitative polygraphic controlled study on efficacy and safety of oral splint devices in tooth-grinding subjects. J Dent Res 2004;83(5):398–403.

163. Okeson JP. The effects of hard and soft occlusal splints on nocturnal bruxism. J Am Dent Assoc 1987;114(6):788–91.

164. Daif ET. Correlation of splint therapy outcome with the electromyography of masticatory muscles in temporomandibular disorder with myofascial pain. Acta Odontol Scand 2012;70(1):72–7.

165. Stapelmann H, Turp JC. The NTI-tss device for the therapy of bruxism, temporomandibular disorders, and headache - where do we stand? A qualitative systematic review of the literature. BMC Oral Health 2008;8:22.

166. Jokstad A, Mo A, Krogstad BS. Clinical comparison between two different splint designs for temporomandibular disorder therapy. Acta Odontol Scand 2005; 63(4):218–26.

167. Jokstad A. The NTI-tss device may be used successfully in the management of bruxism and TMD. Evid Based Dent 2009;10(1):23.

168. Scrivani SJ, Keith DA, Kaban LB. Temporomandibular disorders. N Engl J Med 2008;359(25):2693–705.

169. Al-Ani MZ, Davies SJ, Gray RJ, et al. Stabilisation splint therapy for temporomandibular pain dysfunction syndrome. Cochrane Database Syst Rev 2004;1: CD002778.

170. Fricton J. Myogenous temporomandibular disorders: diagnostic and management considerations. Dent Clin North Am 2007;51(1):61–83, vi.

171. Dao TT, Lavigne GJ. Oral splints: the crutches for temporomandibular disorders and bruxism? Crit Rev Oral Biol Med 1998;9(3):345–61.

172. Fricton J. Current evidence providing clarity in management of temporomandibular disorders: summary of a systematic review of randomized clinical trials for intra-oral appliances and occlusal therapies. J Evid Based Dent Pract 2006; 6(1):48–52.

173. de Felicio CM, de Oliveira MM, da Silva MA. Effects of orofacial myofunctional therapy on temporomandibular disorders. Cranio 2010;28(4):249–59.

174. De Boever JA, Nilner M, Orthlieb JD, et al. Recommendations by the EACD for examination, diagnosis, and management of patients with temporomandibular disorders and orofacial pain by the general dental practitioner. J Orofac Pain 2008;22(3):268–78.

175. Gagnon Y, Mayer P, Morisson F, et al. Aggravation of respiratory disturbances by the use of an occlusal splint in apneic patients: a pilot study. Int J Prosthodont 2004;17(4):447–53.

176. Landry-Schonbeck A, de Grandmont P, Rompre PH, et al. Effect of an adjustable mandibular advancement appliance on sleep bruxism: a crossover sleep laboratory study. Int J Prosthodont 2009;22(3):251–9.

177. Landry ML, Rompre PH, Manzini C, et al. Reduction of sleep bruxism using a mandibular advancement device: an experimental controlled study. Int J Prosthodont 2006;19(6):549–56.

178. Franco L, Rompre PH, de Grandmont P, et al. A mandibular advancement appliance reduces pain and rhythmic masticatory muscle activity in patients with morning headache. J Orofac Pain 2011;25(3):240–9.

179. Martinez-Gomis J, Willaert E, Nogues L, et al. Five years of sleep apnea treatment with a mandibular advancement device. Side effects and technical complications. Angle Orthod 2010;80(1):30–6.

180. de Almeida FR, Lowe AA, Tsuiki S, et al. Long-term compliance and side effects of oral appliances used for the treatment of snoring and obstructive sleep apnea syndrome. J Clin Sleep Med 2005;1(2):143–52.

181. Saletu A, Parapatics S, Saletu B, et al. On the pharmacotherapy of sleep bruxism: placebo-controlled polysomnographic and psychometric studies with clonazepam. Neuropsychobiology 2005;51(4):214–25.

182. Saletu A, Parapatics S, Anderer P, et al. Controlled clinical, polysomnographic and psychometric studies on differences between sleep bruxers and controls and acute effects of clonazepam as compared with placebo. Eur Arch Psychiatry Clin Neurosci 2010;260(2):163–74.

183. Stein DJ, Van Greunen G, Niehaus D. Can bruxism respond to serotonin reuptake inhibitors? J Clin Psychiatry 1998;59(3):133.

184. Brown ES, Hong SC. Antidepressant-induced bruxism successfully treated with gabapentin. J Am Dent Assoc 1999;130(10):1467–9.

185. Mowla A, Sabayan B. Topiramate for bruxism: report of 2 cases. J Clin Psychopharmacol 2010;30(3):346–7.

186. Tan EK, Jankovic J. Treating severe bruxism with botulinum toxin. J Am Dent Assoc 2000;131(2):211–6.

187. Lee SJ, McCall WD Jr, Kim YK, et al. Effect of botulinum toxin injection on nocturnal bruxism: a randomized controlled trial. Am J Phys Med Rehabil 2010;89(1):16–23.

188. Lobbezoo F, Soucy JP, Hartman NG, et al. Effects of the D2 receptor agonist bromocriptine on sleep bruxism: report of two single-patient clinical trials. J Dent Res 1997;76(9):1610–4.

189. Raigrodski AJ, Christensen LV, Mohamed SE, et al. The effect of four-week administration of amitriptyline on sleep bruxism. A double-blind crossover clinical study. Cranio 2001;19(1):21–5.

190. Mohamed SE, Christensen LV, Penchas J. A randomized double-blind clinical trial of the effect of amitriptyline on nocturnal masseteric motor activity (sleep bruxism). Cranio 1997;15(4):326–32.

191. Van der Zaag J, Lobbezoo F, Van der Avoort PG, et al. Effects of pergolide on severe sleep bruxism in a patient experiencing oral implant failure. J Oral Rehabil 2007;34(5):317–22.

192. Kast RE. Tiagabine may reduce bruxism and associated temporomandibular joint pain. Anesth Prog 2005;52(3):102–4.

193. Bostwick JM, Jaffee MS. Buspirone as an antidote to SSRI-induced bruxism in 4 cases. J Clin Psychiatry 1999;60(12):857–60.

Temporomandibular Disorder Pain and Dental Treatment of Obstructive Sleep Apnea

Robert L. Merrill, DDS, MS

KEYWORDS

- Temporomandibular disorder • Dental treatment
- Obstructive sleep apnea

TEMPOROMANDIBULAR DISORDER AND OROFACIAL PAIN

Occasionally, treatment of sleep apnea with mandibular advancement devices (MADs) may be associated with the development of symptoms of temporomandibular disorder (TMD). The clinician needs to determine whether the problem was caused by the MAD or if the problem occurred coincidentally with use of the device. The use of the MAD may cause transient TMD symptoms when the device is first worn, but usually these symptoms resolve within a few days. For those problems that become persistent, treatment of the symptoms should be focused. This article discusses the different types of TMD/orofacial pain (OFP) problems that may occur during treatment of obstructive sleep apnea (OSA) with a MAD. It is critical that the general dentist who is providing dental devices for OSA perform a thorough physical and neurologic assessment of the temporomandibular joint (TMJ) and associated structures before providing such a device so that preexisting problems are identified and discussed with the patient.

ADVERSE EFFECTS OF MADs
Muscle and Joint Tenderness

Use of MADs may be associated with problems such as muscle pain or joint tenderness.[1–4] Jaw tenderness is one of the most common complaints after patients start using the device. It is important to document the presence of muscle or joint tenderness before the delivery of the device. Pain problems including a headache history should be explored in the face-to-face history. The physical examination should

UCLA School of Dentistry, A3-026 CHS, 10833 Le Conte Avenue, Room 10-157, Los Angeles, CA 90095, USA
E-mail address: rmerrill@ucla.edu

Dent Clin N Am 56 (2012) 415–431
doi:10.1016/j.cden.2012.01.004
0011-8532/12/$ – see front matter © 2012 Elsevier Inc. All rights reserved.

include a neurologic examination, evaluation of jaw function, and a palpation examination of the TMJs and cervical and masticatory muscles. A common complaint of patients with OSA is morning headache. However, muscle pain and most particularly myofascial pain (MFP) are frequently associated with or cause headache. A careful palpation examination, performed as part of the initial examination, helps to document preexisting muscle pain and associated headache.

TMJ tenderness can occur with use of MADs. When an appliance holds the jaw in a protrusive position during the night, the joint may become inflamed and tender to palpation. The general term for this condition is capsulitis. Preexisting capsulitis should have been identified before delivery of the appliance, and a definitive diagnosis made at that time. Joint tenderness can be caused by macrotrauma (a sudden injury from a major force) or microtrauma (small repetitive injury) to the joint. Most frequently microtrauma is caused by excessive parafunction both during the day and while sleeping.[5]

Joint Sounds

The presence of joint noises such as clicking or crepitus should also have been determined, diagnosed, and noted in the chart before MAD therapy. Clicking sounds may indicate anterior disk displacement with reduction, whereas crepitus indicates degenerative changes of the condyles. Anterior repositioning is often used to reduce or eliminate clicking. Using a MAD for sleep apnea or snoring may eliminate the TMJ clicking during the night, but the appliance cannot be used in the daytime and the clicking usually returns. Using repositioning appliances 24 hours per day to control or eliminate clicking causes permanent occlusal changes and should not be practiced. Longitudinal studies following clicking over extended periods of time have all shown similar outcomes (ie, the clicks do not get worse and become less of a problem or resolve completely with time).[6–9] Nonpainful clicking does not need to be treated.[10,11]

Joint crepitus (the rubbing sound heard during jaw opening and closing) is often an indication of articular surface remodeling. If the joint is tender to palpation, joint imaging, preferably cone-beam computed tomography (CBCT), should be obtained to determine if degenerative changes have occurred. The combination of crepitus, joint tenderness, and degenerative changes seen on the images is diagnostic of osteoarthritis. If the TMJs are painful at the time of the intake examination, the joint condition should be treated before placement of a MAD because the sleep appliance can aggravate the condition. The clinician should have the patient sign an informed consent form that discusses the current status of the joints and changes that can occur with the use of a MAD. A MAD should be delivered only if the condyles are stable as determined on examination and by palpation and radiographs. Areas of active condylar resorption with pain (eg, osteoarthritis) countermand use of a MAD until the joint inflammation is resolved.[12,13]

Bite Changes

Bite changes have been reported in patients using MADs.[14–16] Commonly, temporary occlusal changes are observed in the morning when the device is removed, requiring the patient to perform some exercises to bring the posterior teeth back together. However, evidence is mounting that long-term use of MADs causes permanent changes in the occlusal relationship. Although patients are given instructions regarding the necessity of performing exercises to bring the posterior teeth back into contact, patients may not perform the exercises as directed and the bite changes can become permanent.[17,18] Changes in the relationship of the maxilla to the mandible have also been documented.[19] These changes represent a gross shift in the jaw relationship in patients with initial class II malocclusions involving a maxillary overjet, or in class III malocclusions in which the anterior incisors are in an edge-to-edge relationship with no maxillary teeth interference with protrusion beyond the edge-to-edge relationship. Although dentofacial and occlusal changes can be attributed to use of an MAD, a recent report shows that long-term use of the CPAP (continuous positive airway pressure) mask without a MAD can also cause dentofacial changes.[20]

Epidemiology of TMD Symptoms and Bite Changes Associated with MAD Use

Increased occurrences of TMD symptoms are not generally associated with use of MADs in the treatment of OSA.[1,21] However, Clark and colleagues[22,23] reported a prevalence estimate of between 10% and 13% of patients using a MAD who developed TMD symptoms that prevented use of the appliance. In addition, it has been reported that the changes became irreversible in 10% of patients using a MAD.[13,24]

Classification of TMD/OFP

Dentists treating snoring and OSA should be familiar with the classification of TMDs and know how to diagnose and treat these problems when they occur. TMDs are broken down into 3 general categories: masticatory muscle disorders, TMJ articular disorders, and inflammatory disorders. The status of the TMJs and musculature must be determined before treatment of OSA with a MAD. The following sections describe the evaluation, diagnosis, and treatment of these disorders.

Masticatory Muscle Disorders

Myalgia
Myalgia is described as a dull, aching, and continuous pain associated with muscle function. The subjective description of the disorder is then confirmed by palpation of the muscles and looking for replication of the pain complaint. If the palpation-induced pain spreads to sites remote from the normal neurosensory distribution of the muscle area, this indicates MFP and not simply myalgia.

MFP
Orofacial MFP has been described in the literature.[8,25] MFP is defined as muscle pain associated with active or latent trigger points that radiate pain to remote sites such as adjacent muscle groups or nonmuscle structures such as the TMJs, sinuses, or teeth. In performing a differential diagnosis for OFP of unclear origin, the clinician should palpate all of the muscle groups that can potentially refer into the area of the pain complaint to see if the source of the pain is coming from the active or latent trigger point. MFP is the great imitator of other painful conditions. The MFP trigger points may also be associated with autonomic features that could confuse and mislead the unwary clinician into thinking the pain was caused by another problem such as neuropathy, dental pain, or a neurovascular disorder when the source of the pain was muscle.[26] **Fig. 1** shows known trigger points in the orofacial and cervical regions that refer pain into the teeth and head.

A clinical examination is accomplished by a thorough muscle palpation of the masticatory and cervical muscle to evaluate for muscle pain. If the patient has muscle pain, finger pressure on the individual muscles causes pain (myalgia) and may generate a referral of pain, as shown in **Fig. 1**. MFP is typically described as continuous, aching, and variable in intensity. MFP can be confirmed by injecting 0.5% procaine or lidocaine without epinephrine into the trigger point or by using ethyl chloride spray while stretching the involved muscle. The pain should decrease by at least 50% to confirm the diagnosis of MFP.[27,28] Myalgia does not refer remotely.

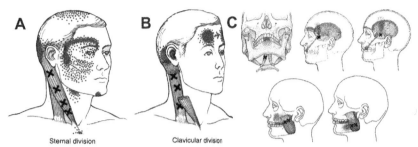

Fig. 1. Myofascial trigger point referral patterns, showing referrals in the orofacial region that are associated with pain and headache. The trigger points are shown as black x's and the referral patterns as the red stippled areas. (*A*) Referrals from the sternal fibers of the sternocleidomastoid muscle. (*B*) Referrals from the clavicular fibers of the sternocleidomastoid muscle. (*C*) Referrals from other masticatory muscles into the teeth. (*From* Simons DG, Travell JG, Simons LS. Travell & Simons' myofascial pain and dysfunction: the trigger point manual. Upper half of body, vol. 1. Baltimore (MD): Lippincott Williams & Wilkins; 1999; with permission.)

Muscle trismus

Muscle trismus or splinting is a protective mechanism that occurs when the muscle fibers shorten and become painful as a protective mechanism limiting movement, or because of trauma. The pain and shortening of the muscle generally avoid repeated trauma. Masticatory muscle splinting is associated with limitation of range of motion and rigidity of the jaw when manipulated. Trismus may be induced as a hysterical reaction caused by psychological distress associated with the pain. Protective splinting is not associated with muscle contraction and increased electromyographic activity when the affected muscle is at rest; consequently, the muscle becomes painful only with function, and splinting increases with stretching of the muscle.[29]

Myositis

Myositis is an inflammatory disorder of muscle caused by infection or trauma within the muscle tissue or by a noninfectious process induced by systemic disease such as polymyositis.[30] Affected pain fibers in the muscles release inflammatory mediators (eg, substance P and calcitonin gene-related peptide [CGRP]), causing the classic signs of inflammation (ie, rubor, dolor, calor, tumor). Characteristically, the myositic muscle is tender to light touch (allodynia), palpation, and functional movement, and, in addition, signs of classic inflammation such as redness and swelling are evident. By comparison, myalgia and MFP are not usually associated with swelling and redness, although pain is induced by palpation and jaw function. Furthermore, in myositis, the inflammation is generalized and the entire muscle is usually affected. In myositis, an increased sedimentation rate is expected, but not in myalgia.

TMJ Articular Disorders

Disk derangements are common in the general population, with prevalence estimates ranging from 40% to 75% of the population.[31] Major trauma also may damage the disk or ligaments (eg, fight, fall, sports injury, oral surgery, or motor vehicle accident), causing the disk to become displaced. Excessive parafunctional activity, such as gum chewing, bruxism, bracing, or clenching, can cause condylar remodeling due to the microtrauma from these parafunctional activities. These behaviors are believed to produce repetitive strain of the joint tissues. In addition, generalized disk ligament laxity may allow the disk to slip forward, leading to disk clicking. Furthermore, disk noises may be an early manifestation of the changes seen in a developing systemic arthritic disease process, altering the condylar form and allowing disk slippage.[32]

The TMD mechanical problems are subcategorized as follows:

1. Disk displacement with reduction: the joint clicks
2. Disk displacement without reduction (close lock): the joint used to click but is now silent
3. Open dislocation
4. Open lock
5. Posterior disk displacement
6. Ankylosis.

Clicking joints

Historically, TMJ clicking was treated with full-time use of an anterior repositioning appliance in an attempt to reduce the anteriorly displaced disk.[33] Although this treatment is still advocated, more recent longitudinal studies suggest that the clicking eventually returns. Further, studies have thrown into doubt the theory that the disk was recaptured.[34–38] However, a subsequent magnetic resonance imaging (MRI) study showed that the displaced disk was not reduced, although the clicking was eliminated.[38] Another study comparing repositioning appliances with flat-plane stabilization appliances for treatment of disk displacements[39] concluded that the repositioning appliance was no better than the stabilization appliances as a treatment option for disk displacement. Treatment of clicking joints is not advocated unless severe pain and dysfunction are associated with the dislocation.[40] In painful clicking and joint dysfunction, the clinician may need to consider fabricating an anterior advancement splint for nighttime use until joint inflammation subsides and the joint adapts to the mechanical dysfunction. Use of a MAD sleep appliance can provide this kind of stabilization. Most anteriorly displaced disks do not cause pain and do not need to be treated.[6,40–42] We do not fully understand why disk slippage occurs but condylar remodeling or stress-induced alterations of the fibrocartilage lining of the joint may predispose the disk to slip forward and occasionally cause pain. In addition, clicks in the joint may not indicate displacement but can be caused by tears or injury to the disk. Joint noises may also be caused by a stick-slip phenomenon, in which the articular surface of the joint is inadequately lubricated, causing the disk to briefly stick to the anterior surface of the eminence. Evidence has accumulated showing that most clicks do not progress to locking, so MRI is not necessary since it would not substantially alter the treatment approach used. In the presence of pain and increased sticking of the disk, CT imaging of the joints should be obtained as part of the diagnostic workup before initiating any joint procedures such as steroid injections or mandibular repositioning.

Locking joints

If the joint is locking and painful, the patient should be referred to a specialist for treatment. The locked joint may need to be manipulated under local anesthetic or an arthrocentesis or lysis and lavage performed to relieve the condition. Stabilization or repositioning appliances may be used after the joint has been unlocked, but these devices cannot be expected to change the status of the lock without some type of joint procedure to remobilize the joint. After a joint procedure, a repositioning appliance may need to be used full time for 1 to 2 weeks to stabilize the joint, allow the inflammation to subside, and discourage the disk from slipping and relocking. This is a short-term expedient and long-term 24-hour-per-day use of this type of splint should be limited because it may cause permanent bite changes.

Inflammatory Joint Disorders

Although several monoarthritic and polyarthritic conditions can affect the TMJs, this article focuses only on the most likely conditions to be confronted by a general dentist who is treating OSA (ie, capsulitis, osteoarthritis, and rheumatoid arthritis). TMJ arthritis is not a unified disorder. Several inflammatory conditions can affect the TMJ but many are obscure and not often seen; however, most show overlapping clinical symptoms. The diagnosis of many inflammatory joint disorders is made based on the clinical signs and radiological and laboratory findings. However, most TMJ arthritis seen in a clinical setting is degenerative or osteoarthritic in nature and is not reflective of systemic disease. The diagnosis of osteoarthritis is made from the history, clinical signs, and symptoms rather than from laboratory findings. The TMJ apparatus, including disk function, is susceptible to arthritic changes, and pain may precede the degenerative changes.

Arthralgia/capsulitis

Inflammatory conditions of the TMJs are categorized as localized arthralgia (capsulitis), localized arthritis, and polyarthritis involving the TMJs. Localized and specific joint pain or tenderness is called arthralgia or capsulitis. These terms are used after tenderness has been confirmed with palpation. Arthralgia is used to describe palpable joint pain with no evidence of crepitus or osseous changes on the radiographs. The terms retrodiscitis or synovitis are occasionally used when the dorsal aspect of the TMJ capsule is tender to palpation, but these terms imply a diagnosis that can be made only through biopsy evaluation of the tissue.

The most important cause of arthralgia is trauma, either from external injury or traumatic parafunction. Trauma induces a local inflammation in the joint that is associated with inflammatory mediators released into the joint space. The mediators cause sensitization of the joint nociceptors, joint swelling, warmth, and pain. The inflammatory response causes alterations of the soft and hard tissues in the joint, leading to bony remodeling. Other causes of joint pain may be infection or a localized manifestation of a polyarthritic disorder.

Trauma may induce arthritis when the intra-articular soft tissues are compressed from trauma. The mandible may deviate to the side of the injury in the intercuspal position as a result of damage to the joint structure, muscle guarding, or swelling of the involved joint. The opening is restricted by inflammation in the joint and by guarding and trismus of the masticatory muscles. This situation often causes a shift in muscle-guided closing and opening positions of the jaw. If the joint is edematous, there may be no tooth-to-tooth contacts on the ipsilateral side.

The pain is described as aching in the preauricular area and often in the ear itself. It is aggravated by jaw function such as chewing, talking, opening wide, and lateral movements of the jaw. Palpation of the lateral and dorsal capsules of the joints replicates the pain. In addition, pain is caused by manually loading the joint, pushing the condyle up and back in the fossa, or by having the patient bite on a tongue blade placed between the posterior teeth on the opposite side. Wearing a MAD may cause capsulitis in some patients, particularly when the appliance is removed in the morning and the patient clenches the jaw to bring the posterior teeth into contact. Because capsulitis represents a localized inflammation of the capsule and retrodiscal tissues, the condition needs to be treated to lessen the likelihood that the continuation of joint inflammation leads to degenerative joint changes. Capsulitis is not seen with radiographic examination unless it is severe and associated with inflammatory mediated joint effusion. Excessive loading of the joints is associated with free radical production and release of inflammatory neuropeptides such as substance P and CGRP, which cause neurogenic inflammation and swelling in the joints.[34,43,44] This process leads to breakdown of the TMJ and osteoarthritis.

Osteoarthritis

As mentioned earlier, TMJ osteoarthritis is one of the most common joint problems seen in the population that is being treated for OSA with a dental device. The prevalence of osteoarthritis increases with age, and this is the same age group in which the prevalence of OSA is more likely to occur. Osteoarthritis of the TMJ may be limited to 1 joint (monoarticular) or both (diarticular). The monoarticular form is more likely a result of trauma to the joint, whereas bilateral changes are more often caused by systemic factors or traumatic parafunctional activity. In addition, a previous nonreducing disk displacement may lead to degenerative changes in the affected joint.[45]

The criteria for making a diagnosis of osteoarthritis are (1) palpable joint pain, (2) crepitus, and (3) radiological evidence of joint degeneration. Most arthritic TMJs have crepitant noises with joint movement. The presence of osteoarthritis needs to be ascertained in the initial examination. In addition, degenerative changes and crepitus may be present without pain. The degenerative changes could make the TMJ more susceptible to abnormal stresses with the use of a MAD.

If no pain is found on palpation of the joints but crepitus is present, or if the joint is palpably tender and crepitant, further evaluation with joint radiographs is warranted. Usually, TMJ osteoarthritis does not manifest swelling or redness because the magnitude of any inflammation is small when compared with the systemic autoimmune inflammatory disorders. Nevertheless, an acute inflammation of an arthritic joint may be associated with swelling and subsequent loss of posterior occlusal contacts on the side of the swelling. Once the joint has been treated appropriately, the occlusal contacts normalize.

There are 2 major types of traumatic injuries that induce local osteoarthritis: macrotrauma, which is caused by an external sharp force against the jaw and microtrauma as a result of repeated parafunctional activity. Another less recognized form of trauma leading to TMJ osteoarthritis under conditions of normal function occurs when a patient has had a previous disk derangement (displacement without reduction), causing joint degeneration probably as a result of loss of the disk, the shock absorber of the joint.[46] As discussed earlier for capsulitis, the neurogenic inflammatory process related to pain and swelling in the TMJ also leads to both soft tissue and bony degeneration of the TMJs.

There are no biologic markers for osteoarthritis that can be determined in laboratory tests, so, as noted earlier, the diagnosis relies on palpation to confirm the pain is of joint origin, auscultation of joint noises, and radiographs (CBCT) (**Fig. 2**) of the TMJ and other joints to confirm if the arthritic remodeling process is present.

Rheumatoid arthritis

Rheumatoid arthritis is an autoimmune disorder that causes the destruction of the patient's own tissues. It starts as an inflammatory soft tissue disease, which may not show radiographic evidence of bony degeneration until the later stages of the disease. This form of arthritis is not as common as osteoarthritis but is seen frequently in older patients, who also may have OSA. The antigenic trigger of rheumatoid arthritis is the synovial tissues and not the articular surface of joint, but as the destruction of the synovia progresses, the entire joint is affected. Typically, rheumatoid arthritis in the

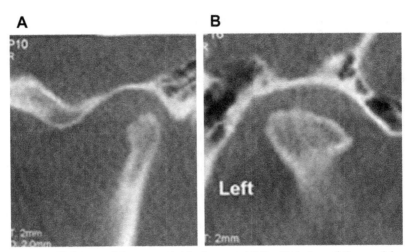

Fig. 2. CBCT of left TMJ with osteoarthritic changes. (*A*) Sagittal view of the condyle, with obvious flattening and roughness of the articular surface. (*B*) Coronal view of the condyle, with flattening particularly obvious on the lateral pole of the condyle.

TMJ is also accompanied by pain in other joints, and the older patient may present with joint disfigurement. Rheumatoid patients present with restricted opening and a progressive anterior open bite. The patient should be under the care of a rheumatologist and a referral should be made if the disease is suspected. Use of a MAD for sleep apnea is problematic because the forces of the appliance could adversely affect the joint. Laboratory tests are performed to look for positive rheumatoid factor (RF) or anti-CCP (anticyclic citrullinated peptide antibody). These tests are positive in 70% of rheumatoid patients but if the RF factor is positive, the anti-CCP test does not give any additional useful information.

THE TMD EXAMINATION AND DIAGNOSIS

There are several parts of the physical examination for the evaluation of a patient with sleep apnea. This article focuses on the OFP examination. The data gleaned from this examination should identify potential problems that may develop or be aggravated when a patient is using a MAD. The overall OFP examination is broken down into 5 parts: (1) the chief complaint and history of present illness, (2) the cranial nerve examination, (3) the stomatognathic examination, (4) the palpation examination, and (5) other examinations and tests.

Chief Complaint and History of Present Illness

The chief complaint and history of present illness as well as a review of current pain symptoms include onset, quality, location, temporal pattern, course of pain over a 24-hour period, modifying factors, and impact of the pain. Because headache is often a symptom of sleep apnea, the pain history should also include a detailed headache history. It is important in reviewing the headache history to ask about headache accompaniments such as sensitivity to light and sound, presence of nausea (symptoms of migraine), and autonomic features that occur with the headache such as nasal congestion, conjunctival injection, ptosis, and tearing (symptoms of the autonomic cephalalgias).[47] In addition, the clinician should always be aware that not all headaches are benign or primary headache disorders. Important red flags always to consider when evaluating patient are:

1. A new headache that is different from previous headaches
2. The worst ever headache
3. A headache that gets worse when the patient lies down
4. A headache that reaches maximum intensity within seconds to a few minutes
5. A headache associated with neurologic symptoms such as numbness, loss of vision, confusion, and loss of consciousness.

Cranial Nerve Examination

The cranial nerve screening examination evaluates the gross function of the cranial nerves. This examination is performed to help rule out an intracranial or neuropathic source of the pain. Expanding intracranial lesions are space occupying and begin to put pressure on structures and nerves that cause pain or impair function (**Table 1**).

The Stomatognathic Examination

The stomatognathic examination evaluates the general function of the jaw, including the range of comfort opening, active opening, and passive stretch opening, as well as the extent of lateral jaw movements and whether the opening path deviates or

Table 1
Cranial nerves and function. The cranial nerve examination should be part of the OFP and sleep examination. A demonstration of the examination can be viewed at http://www.neuroexam.com

Cranial Nerve	Name	Function
I	Olfactory	Smells
II	Optic	Sees
III	Occulomotor	Extraocular eye movements, constricts pupils
IV	Trochlear	Extraocular eye movement (looks to nose and down)
V	Trigeminal	Sensory to face, motor to muscles of mastication
VI	Abducens	Extraocular eye movement (looks to side)
VII	Facial	Motor for facial muscles of expression, sudomotor for crying and spitting, visceral sensory for taste from two-thirds of lateral border of tongue, somatic sensory to anterior wall of external auditory meatus
VIII	Vestibulocochlear	Hearing and balance
IX	Glossopharyngeal	Elevates palate, parotid salivation, somatic sensory from middle ear, external auditory meatus, pharynx and posterior one-third of tongue. Taste from posterior one-third of tongue, chemoreceptors, and baroreceptors of carotid body
X	Vagus	Swallows, parasympathetic enervation to heart lungs, digestive tract, sensation from pharynx, meninges and external auditory meatus, tastes from epiglottis and pharynx, chemoreceptors and baroreceptors of aortic arch
XI	Accessory	Turns head (sternocleidomastoid muscle) and shrugs shoulders (trapezius muscle)
XII	Hypoglossal	Intrinsic muscles of tongue. Sticks out the tongue

deflects during opening. The examination also determines the presence of joint noises, both crepitus and clicking, and whether there are anomalies in the tooth-to-tooth contacts. These deviations from normal should be charted carefully because wearing a MAD may change the tooth-to-tooth contacts and jaw relationships. Severity of tooth wear and tongue/cheek ridging are also charted.

The Palpation Examination

The palpation examination evaluates the TMJs and muscles for pain by separately palpating each joint and muscle to determine the presence of pain and possible referral patterns from the muscles. In this part of the examination, the examiner is trying to replicate the patient's pain complaint. The dorsal and lateral poles of each condyle are palpated separately and the patient is asked if it is painful. Each of the masticatory muscles is palpated separately, and during the palpation the patient is asked how severe the pain is on a scale of 0 to 3 and if the pain is radiating away from the palpation site. This is an important distinction that helps to differentiate myalgia from MFP. As shown in **Fig. 3**, each muscle is palpated separately with 1 finger that rubs across the muscle fiber at the palpation site with a pressure of approximately 1.8 to 2.3 kg (4 to 5 pounds). This test allows a myofascial trigger point to develop the characteristic radiation pattern for that muscle (**Fig. 4**).

TREATING TMD PROBLEMS DURING MAD THERAPY FOR OSA

Treatment of TMD is based on the type of problem that has occurred. In addition to joint pain, the most common problems associated with TMDs are myalgia and MFP. As discussed earlier, it is important to distinguish between the 2 disorders in the examination by looking for referral pain and radiation of tenderness from the palpated tender areas of the muscles. In addition, changes in occlusion that may occur during the use of a MAD need to be addressed early in the MAD treatment because changes that have been ignored or unevaluated for weeks to months are most likely irreversible with simple exercises, and more involved dental restorative procedures or orthodontics may be needed to resolve the problem.[48,49]

Capsulitis (The Tender Joint)

If the patient is complaining of pain in the TMJs and the joints are tender to palpation, the patient should be instructed to go on a soft diet, avoiding chewing any hard foods,

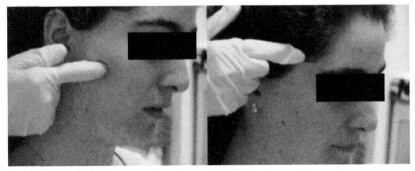

Fig. 3. Muscle palpation examination showing the palpation of the muscles using a single digit and palpating each muscle individually. This test is performed to allow a myofascial trigger point, if present, to develop and radiate.

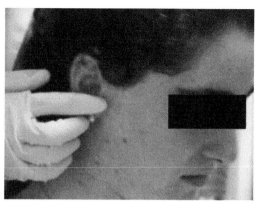

Fig. 4. Joint palpation is performed by pushing on the lateral and dorsal aspects of the TMJ.

cutting food (eg, apples) into small bites, and steaming vegetables. We may think of salads as soft but they usually require a lot of chewing, so the patient should be wary of eating chewy salads until the pain resolves. The patient also should be instructed to reduce jaw function by not chewing gum. In addition, the patient should be instructed to use moist heat on the jaw 2 to 3 times per day. This task can be achieved by folding a bath towel into a square, wetting the towel, wringing the excess water out, placing the towel in a plastic bag, and heating it in a microwave oven for 5 minutes. The towel is then removed from the microwave oven and plastic bag and covered with a dry towel. This hot packet is then placed over the painful joint and held for about 10 minutes. This process should be repeated 2 to 3 times per day (**Fig. 5**).

Antiinflammatory medications such as naproxen (Naprosyn 500 mg taken twice per day or 2 Aleve twice per day) should be prescribed or recommended. If ibuprofen is to be used, a prescription should be written for 600-mg to 800-mg tablets, with instructions to take 1 tablet 3 times per day. These medications should be taken with food. If the patient has a history of stomach irritation such as gastroesophageal reflux disease

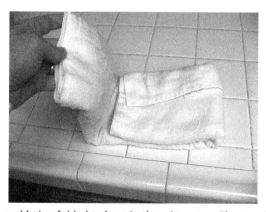

Fig. 5. Wet bath towel being folded to heat in the microwave. The towel should be placed in a plastic bag and then heated in the microwave for 5 minutes. After being removed from the microwave, the towel is removed from the plastic bag and covered with a dry towel before placing on the jaw.

or reflux, they can take 20 mg of omeprazole or lansoprazole per day to reduce acidity. If the nonsteroidal antiinflammatory drug is not helpful, a prescription for a methylprednisolone (Medrol) dose pack may be helpful in decreasing the inflammation. For an acutely painful joint, if these procedures are not helping, the patient should be referred to an OFP specialist or oral surgeon, who can inject a steroid or hyaluronic acid into the joint.

In addition to decreasing joint loading by softening the diet, the patient should be instructed to use what has been termed a hinge axis exercise to rotate the condyles in the fossae without opening wide enough to cause translation of the condyles down the eminence. This exercise is performed by having the patient quickly open and close the jaw about a finger width without tapping the teeth in the close position. The procedure is to be performed 10 times consecutively and this process should be repeated several times through the waking day. The movement stimulates the production of synovial fluid, lubricating the joint and helping to decrease inflammation.

The oral appliance needs to be reevaluated to see if it is advancing the jaw too much. The clinician should achieve a balance between the amount of advancement versus the increase in vertical. Studies have shown that increasing the vertical is as important as mandibular advancement.[21] Increasing the vertical is usually less irritating to the TMJ than advancing the mandible.

Anterior Disk Displacement with Reduction (The Clicking Joint)

The presence of a click should have been determined and documented before treatment with a MAD. The differential diagnosis for clicking includes anterior disk displacement with reduction, joint remodeling as a result of mechanical stress to the joint, and osteoarthritis. Joint imaging is not needed if there is no associated pain or crepitus. Clicking as a result of anterior disk displacement does not usually occur with the use of a MAD because the mandibular advancement is expected to reduce the likelihood of the disk slipping anteriorly. However, mandibular advancement and the irritation of the appliance may exacerbate bruxism during the night, with consequent development of clicking associated with the increased working of the joints. In addition, heavy parafunction at night can cause a stick-slip phenomenon, in which the excessive loading of the joint pushes out the lubricating synovial fluid from between the eminence and the disk, causing the disk to stick to the eminence and subsequently reduce and click when the space is relubricated.

Anterior Disk Displacement Without Reduction (The Locked Joint)

Patients who have developed a nonreducing anterior displacement should be seen by an OFP specialists or an oral surgeon who has had experience in dealing with this problem. Treatment involves joint manipulation of the anesthetized joint, arthrocentesis, and pumping of the joint, or arthroscopic surgery. Open joint surgery is rarely needed, and although there are several case series in the literature describing relative success for surgical procedures to remove the disk, plicate the posterior ligament, and suture or staple the disk in place, there are no good prospective, randomized, double-blind clinical trials that show benefit from these procedures.[50]

MYOGENOUS PAIN

Masticatory and cervical muscle tenderness is the most common problem associated with TMD. Treatment requires the use of physical therapy, physical medicine techniques, and possibly medication management to optimize the treatment. The patient who develops muscle tenderness while using a MAD should be given instructions for

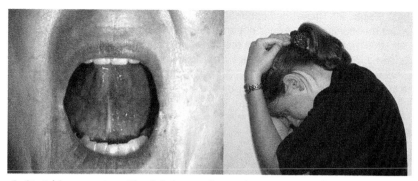

Fig. 6. Stretching exercises. The left image shows the tongue on the palate behind the upper front teeth and the jaw being stretched to the point at which the tongue would be pulled off the palate if the patient opened wider. The right image shows the patient stretching the posterior neck muscles that are often painful in association with the jaw muscles.

stretching the masticatory muscles during the day. This process should start after removal of the MAD and the exercises to reestablish posterior tooth-to-tooth contacts. The patient should be instructed to stretch the jaw by placing the tongue on the palate behind the upper front teeth and stretching open as far as they can stretch without pulling the tongue off of the palate (**Fig. 6**). The stretch is held for 6 seconds, repeated 6 times, and the process is repeated 6 times per day. This exercise stretches the masseter, medial pterygoid, and temporalis muscles. If the muscles are severely tender, the patient should use moist heat for 5 minutes before the stretching exercises and then ice to cool down the muscles for 5 minutes after the stretching.

The patient should also be instructed to assume a jaw rest position during the day. This practice helps the patient to avoid daytime clenching that can keep the muscles tender. The patient is instructed to place the tongue on the palate similar to the jaw position assumed for the stretch in **Fig. 6**, but the lips are brought together and the teeth kept slightly apart. The patient is also instructed to breathe through the nose in this position. This rest position helps to reduce masseter, medial pterygoid, and temporalis muscle activity.

ADJUNCTIVE MEDICATIONS

In addition to the medications discussed earlier, other classes of medications can be helpful in mediating the pain. Muscle relaxants can be a helpful addition to treating the

Table 2
Muscle relaxants

Generic	Proprietary	Dose
Cyclobenzaprine	Flexeril	10 mg at bedtime
Tizanidine	Zanaflex	2–4 mg (dosed 3 times a day up to 16 mg)
Baclofen	Lioresal	5–10 (dosed 3 times a day up to 80 mg)
Metaxalone	Skelaxin	800 mg 3 to 4 times a day
Methocarbamol	Robaxin	500–750 mg (1500 mg 4 times a day)
Soma	Carisoprodol	250–350 mg 3 times a day. Use for maximum of 2 weeks

jaw pain (**Table 2**). These medications individually are associated with side effects. The exact mechanism of action is not understood. All of the medications cause sedation, and this may be the main effect they have on muscle activity. Some medications may affect blood pressure and heart rate (tizanidine and cyclobenzaprine) or can cause weight gain (cyclobenzaprine). Carisoprodol is metabolized to meprobamate, which is a major tranquilizer and is addictive.

SUMMARY

This article discusses the evaluation and treatment of TMJ problems from the perspective of symptoms that may be associated with the use of a MAD for treating OSA. A thorough head and neck examination should be performed before initiating appliance therapy for sleep, and any indications of joint dysfunction, pain in joints or muscles, and bite discrepancies should be documented, discussed with the patient, and, if need be, treated before initiating therapy with a MAD. When pain occurs after the patient has started wearing the appliance, procedures for evaluating and treating the pain are discussed. Usually, if pain develops with initial use of the appliance, it is temporary, but the stretching exercises for muscle pain and the hinge axis movement for joint pain help to ameliorate it. If the pain becomes more persistent, the patient should be advised to discontinue use of the appliance while pain management procedures are put in place. The appliance should be reassessed to see if the horizontal advancement can be reduced and the vertical opening can be increased. Often, a change of 1 mm can make a significant change to the pain. Patients who have significant painful arthritic changes in the joints may not be able to wear an appliance until the joint inflammation is controlled by a joint procedure, such as arthrocentesis, lysis and lavage, or arthroscopy. This procedure should be performed only by an OFP specialist or an oral surgeon who has experience in managing acute joint problems.

REFERENCES

1. Hoekema A, Stegenga B, De Bont LG. Efficacy and co-morbidity of oral appliances in the treatment of obstructive sleep apnea-hypopnea: a systematic review. Crit Rev Oral Biol Med 2004;15(3):137–55.
2. Sutherland K, Cistulli P. Mandibular advancement splints for the treatment of sleep apnea syndrome. Swiss Med Wkly 2011;141:w13276.
3. Ferguson KA, Cartwright R, Rogers R, et al. Oral appliances for snoring and obstructive sleep apnea: a review. Sleep 2006;29(2):244–62.
4. Hammond RJ, Gotsopoulos H, Shen G, et al. A follow-up study of dental and skeletal changes associated with mandibular advancement splint use in obstructive sleep apnea. Am J Orthod Dentofacial Orthop 2007;132(6):806–14.
5. Clark GT, Sakai S, Merrill R, et al. Cross-correlation between stress, pain, physical activity, and temporalis muscle EMG in tension-type headache. Cephalalgia 1995;15(6):511–8 [discussion: 451].
6. Mejersjo C, Carlsson GE. Long-term results of treatment for temporomandibular joint pain-dysfunction. J Prosthet Dent 1983;49:809–15.
7. Greene CS, Laskin DM. Long-term evaluation of conservative treatment for myofascial pain-dysfunction syndrome. J Am Dent Assoc 1974;89:1365–8.
8. Greene CS, Laskin DM. Long-term evaluation of treatment for myofascial pain-dysfunction syndrome: a comparative analysis. J Am Dent Assoc 1983;107:235–8.

9. Magnusson T, Carlsson GE, Egermark I. Changes in subjective symptoms of cra-niomandibular disorders in children and adolescents during a 10 year period. J Orofac Pain 1993;7:76–82.

10. Barghan S, Merrill R, Tetradis S. Cone beam computed tomography imaging in the evaluation of the temporomandibular joint. J Calif Dent Assoc 2010;38(1): 33–9.

11. Clark GT, Merrill RL. The diagnosis and treatment of masticatory muscle pain and dysfunction. In: Sarnat BG, Laskin D, editors. The temporomandibular joint: a bio-logic basis for clinical practice. 4th edition. Philadelphia: W.B. Saunders, Publisher; 1991. Chapter 21.

12. Kobayashi T, Izumi N, Kojima T, et al. Progressive condylar resorption after mandibular advancement. Br J Oral Maxillofac Surg 2011. [Epub ahead of print].

13. Clark GT. Mandibular advancement devices and sleep disordered breathing. Sleep Med Rev 1998;2(3):163–74.

14. Rose EC, Staats R, Virchow C Jr, et al. Occlusal and skeletal effects of an oral appliance in the treatment of obstructive sleep apnea. Chest 2002;122(3):871–7.

15. Marklund M. Predictors of long-term orthodontic side effects from mandibular advancement devices in patients with snoring and obstructive sleep apnea. Am J Orthod Dentofacial Orthop 2006;129(2):214–21.

16. Otsuka R, Almeida FR, Lowe AA. The effects of oral appliance therapy on occlusal function in patients with obstructive sleep apnea: a short-term prospec-tive study. Am J Orthod Dentofacial Orthop 2007;131(2):176–83.

17. Ueda H, Almeida FR, Lowe AA, et al. Changes in occlusal contact area during oral appliance therapy assessed on study models. Angle Orthod 2008;78(5): 866–72.

18. Ueda H, Almeida FR, Chen H, et al. Effect of 2 jaw exercises on occlusal function in patients with obstructive sleep apnea during oral appliance therapy: a random-ized controlled trial. Am J Orthod Dentofacial Orthop 2009;135(4):430 e431–7 [discussion: 430–1].

19. Tsuiki S, Ryan CF, Lowe AA, et al. Functional contribution of mandibular advance-ment to awake upper airway patency in obstructive sleep apnea. Sleep Breath 2007;11(4):245–51.

20. Tsuda H, Almeida FR, Tsuda T, et al. Craniofacial changes after 2 years of nasal continuous positive airway pressure use in patients with obstructive sleep apnea. Chest 2010;138:870–4.

21. de Almeida FR, Bittencourt LR, de Almeida CI, et al. Effects of mandibular posture on obstructive sleep apnea severity and the temporomandibular joint in patients fitted with an oral appliance. Sleep 2002;25(5):507–13.

22. Clark GT, Arand D, Chung E, et al. Effect of anterior mandibular positioning on obstructive sleep apnea. Am Rev Respir Dis 1993;147(3):624–9.

23. Clark GT, Kobayashi H, Freymiller E. Mandibular advancement and sleep disor-dered breathing. CDA J 1996;24(4):49–61.

24. Petit FX, Pepin JL, Bettega G, et al. Mandibular advancement devices: rate of contraindications in 100 consecutive obstructive sleep apnea patients. Am J Respir Crit Care Med 2002;166(3):274–8.

25. Laskin DM, Greene CS, Hylander WL, editors. TMDs: an evidence-based approach to diagnosis and treatment. Chicago: Quintessence Publishing; 2006.

26. Part 2, Head and neck pain. In: Simons DG, Travell JG, Simons LS, editors. Travell & Simons' myofascial pain and dysfunction: the trigger point manual, vol. 1. Upper half of body. 2nd edition. Baltimore (MD): Lippincott Williams & Wilkins; 1999. p. 237–77. Chapter 5.

27. Graff-Radford SB. Myofascial trigger points: their importance and diagnosis in the dental office. J Dent Assoc S Afr 1984;39:249–53.

28. Graff-Radford SB. Myofascial pain: diagnosis and management. Curr Pain Headache Rep 2004;8(6):463–7.

29. Clark GT, Seligman DA, Solberg WK, et al. Guidelines for the treatment of temporomandibular disorders. J Craniomandib Disord 1990;4(2):80–8.

30. Clark GT, Seligman DA, Solberg WK, et al. Guidelines for the examination and diagnosis of temporomandibular disorders. J Craniomandib Disord 1989;3(1):7–14.

31. Dworkin SF, LeResche L. Research diagnostic criteria for temporomandibular disorders: review, criteria, examinations and specifications, critique. J Craniomandib Disord 1992;6(4):301–55.

32. Clark GT, Merrill RL. The diagnosis and treatment of internal derangements. In: Sarnat BG, Laskin D, editors. The temporomandibular joint: a biologic basis for clinical practice. 4th edition. Philadelphia: W.B. Saunders, Publisher; 1991. Chapter 23.

33. Farrar WB. Diagnosis and treatment of anterior dislocation of the articular disc. N Y J Dent 1971;41(10):348–51.

34. Clark GT. A critical evaluation of orthopedic interocclusal appliance therapy: design, theory and overall effectiveness. J Am Dent Assoc 1984;108:359–62.

35. Okeson JP. Long-term treatment of disk-interference disorders of the temporomandibular joint with anterior repositioning occlusal splints. J Prosthet Dent 1988;60(5):611–6.

36. Lundh H, Westesson PL, Kopp S, et al. Anterior repositioning splint in the treatment of temporomandibular joints with reciprocal clicking: comparison with a flat occlusal splint and an untreated control group. Oral Surg Oral Med Oral Pathol 1985;60(2):131–6.

37. Lundh H, Westesson PL. Long-term follow-up after occlusal treatment to correct abnormal temporomandibular joint disk position. Oral Surg Oral Med Oral Pathol 1989;67(1):2–10.

38. Tallents RH, Katzberg RW, Macher DJ, et al. Use of protrusive splint therapy in anterior disk displacement of the temporomandibular joint: a 1- to 3-year follow-up. J Prosthet Dent 1990;63(3):336–41.

39. Tecco S, Festa F, Salini V, et al. Treatment of joint pain and joint noises associated with a recent TMJ internal derangement: a comparison of an anterior repositioning splint, a full-arch maxillary stabilization splint, and an untreated control group. Cranio 2004;22(3):209–19.

40. De Leeuw R, editor. Orofacial pain; guidelines for assessment, diagnosis, and management. 4th edition. Hanover Park (IL): Quintessence Books; 2008.

41. Clark GT. Treatment of jaw clicking with temporomandibular repositioning: analysis of 25 cases. J Craniomandibular Pract 1984;2:263–70.

42. Seligman DA, Pullinger AG, Solberg WK. The prevalence of dental attrition and its association with factors of age, gender, occlusion, and TMJ symptomatology. J Dent Res 1988;67(10):1323–33.

43. Fukuoka Y, Hagihara M, Nagatsu T, et al. The relationship between collagen metabolism and temporomandibular joint osteoarthrosis in mice. J Oral Maxillofac Surg 1993;51(3):288–91.

44. Hutchins B, Patel H, Spears R. Attenuation of pro-inflammatory neuropeptide levels produced by a cyclooxygenase-2 inhibitor in an animal model of chronic temporomandibular joint inflammation. J Orofac Pain 2002;16(4):312–6.

45. Pullinger AG, Seligman DA. Multifactorial analysis of differences in temporomandibular joint hard tissue anatomic relationships between disk displacement with and without reduction in women. J Prosthet Dent 2001;86(4):407–19.

46. Sylvester DC, Exss E, Marholz C, et al. Association between disk position and degenerative bone changes of the temporomandibular joints: an imaging study in subjects with TMD. Cranio 2011;29(2):117–26.

47. Silberstein SD, Lipton RB, Dodick D, et al. In: Wolff's headache and other head pain. 8th edition. Oxford (UK); New York: Oxford University Press; 2008. p. 379–430. Chapter 14.

48. Almeida FR, Lowe AA, Sung JO, et al. Long-term sequellae of oral appliance therapy in obstructive sleep apnea patients: part 1. Cephalometric analysis. Am J Orthod Dentofacial Orthop 2006;129(2):195–204.

49. Almeida FR, Lowe AA, Otsuka R, et al. Long-term sequellae of oral appliance therapy in obstructive sleep apnea patients: part 2. Study-model analysis. Am J Orthod Dentofacial Orthop 2006;129(2):205–13.

50. Laskin DM. Surgical management of internal derangements. In: Laskin D, Greene CS, Hylander WL, editors. TMDs: an evidence-based approach to diagnosis and treatment. Chicago: Quintessence Publishing; 2006. p. 469–81.

Effectiveness and Outcome of Oral Appliance Therapy

Benjamin T. Pliska, DDS, MS, FRCD(C)*, Fernanda Almeida, DDS, PhD

KEYWORDS

- Oral appliances therapy • Obstructive sleep apnea
- Continuous positive airway pressure
- Mandibular advancement splints

Oral appliances (OAs) are indicated as a primary treatment option for snoring and mild to moderate obstructive sleep apnea (OSA)[1] and are also being implemented as a noninvasive alternative for patients with severe OSA who are unwilling or unable to tolerate continuous positive airway pressure (CPAP) for the management of their disease. CPAP is an effective treatment for the management of sleep-disordered breathing in both adults and children but has low adherence rates. Therefore, OAs play an important role in the therapy for patients with OSA. There is continued emergence of studies demonstrating the ability of OAs to eliminate or significantly reduce the symptoms of OSA and produce a measurable influence on the long-term health effects of the disease. Most studies have evaluated one type of OA, mandibular advancement splints (MAS). Therefore, this article describes the effectiveness and outcomes of MAS.

Over the past decade, several randomized controlled clinical trials have been conducted comparing the effects of MAS against both placebo devices[2-10] and CPAP.[2,3,11-22] The efficacy of MAS has been reviewed previously, including a Cochrane review[23] and a practice parameter update by the American Academy of Sleep Medicine[1]; all together, there is a considerable body of evidence toward the efficacy of MAS in the treatment of OSA. To summarize the efficacy studies, in randomized controlled trials comparing MAS with placebo, MAS have been shown to significantly improve objective sleep measurements, such as the apnea-hypopnea index (AHI), arousal index, snoring, and in some but not all studies, arterial oxygen desaturation. MAS have also been shown to significantly improve subjective and objective measurements of sleepiness, quality of life, and 24-hour blood pressure measurement devices.[2-10] A variety of randomized controlled trials have compared the efficacy of MAS with CPAP.[2,3,11-18] According to

Department of Oral Health Sciences, University of British Columbia, 2199 Wesbrook Mall, Vancouver, British Columbia V6T 1Z3, Canada
* Corresponding author.
E-mail address: pliska@dentistry.ubc.ca

Dent Clin N Am 56 (2012) 433–444
doi:10.1016/j.cden.2012.02.003   **dental.theclinics.com**

these trials, both CPAP and MAS improved objective sleep measurements, such as AHI, arousal index, and minimum arterial oxygen saturation. Although CPAP and MAS have similar improvements in cardiovascular outcomes and inflammatory markers,[24] the magnitude of improvements in AHI and oxygen saturation was significantly greater with CPAP. This contradiction may likely be related to a higher adherence to MAS compared with CPAP in terms of hours per night and nights per week of usage.[3] **Table 1** summarizes the outcomes of the most recent studies.

MAS increase the upper airway by preventing the tongue and soft tissues of the throat from collapsing into the pharynx while holding the mandible and attached soft tissues, including the tongue base forward, which enlarges the upper airway dimensions by specifically increasing the lateral dimensions of the velopharynx.[25]

FACTORS IMPACTING THE EFFECTIVENESS OF OSA TREATMENT WITH MAS
Adherence

Adherence has been defined by the World Health Organization as "the extent to which a person's behavior – taking medications, following a diet, and/or executing lifestyle changes, such as using CPAP or MAS every night – correspond with agreed recommendations from a heath care provider."[26] Poor adherence to long-term treatment is often a problem faced by health professionals, and unfortunately there is a paucity of specific training in adherence management for practitioners. To improve adherence, it is known that a patient-centered treatment approach is crucial and patient preferences and lifestyle has to be taken into account. The consequences of a nontailored method with poor patient adherence are related to poor health outcomes and increased health care costs.

The effectiveness of mandibular advancement device (MAD) therapy depends on patient adherence to wear the device comfortably, and appliances that are custom made and adjustable have been found to be more effective than the fixed, thermoplastic-type appliances.[27,28] Vanderveken and collaborators[27] have shown that prefabricated, off-the-shelf appliances are less effective and less accepted by patients and, therefore, should not be used either as a therapeutic option or as a screening tool to predict MAS responders.

An area where MAS are described to excel compared with CPAP is the rate of patient adherence to the prescribed treatment regimen. Adherence is usually measured subjectively, and self-reported compliance with appliance use has been reported to be as high as 96% in patients using MAS for more than 75% of nights and 80% in patients using MAD more than 75% of each night.[12] The bias that can accompany self-reported adherence is highlighted by one study whereby a compliance monitor indicated that the MAD was worn for a mean of 6.8 hours per night.[29]

According to randomized controlled trials, CPAP therapy is consistently more effective at reducing sleep-disordered breathing events, but patients tolerate MAS better.[2,3,11–18] The superior patient satisfaction associated with the use of MAS reflects the relative simplicity and convenience of this form of treatment. Despite residual apneas with MAS, or a higher efficacy rate of CPAP in reducing the AHI, the similarities in treatment outcomes have been previously hypothesized to be related to the numbers of hours per night of use. MAS used for prolonged hours with partial efficacy may result in similar outcomes compared with CPAP being fully effective for only part of the night. A patient-tailored treatment is synonymous with good medicine, and life-long therapies are dependent on patients' cooperation and adherence. It is important to include patients in the decision of their treatment and offer more than

Table 1
Summary of some recent randomized controlled trials comparing MAS with CPAP

Author, Year, Reference Number of Patients	Measurements	Significant Changes Compared with Baseline	Significant Changes Compared with CPAP	Patients Who Preferred a Treatment (%)
Hoekema et al,[22] 2007 N = 20	PSG ESS Driving performance	MAS and CPAP improved AHI, min SaO2 Both improved ESS CPAP and MAS improved	MAS = CPAP MAS = CPAP MAS = CPAP	N/A Parallel study
Hoekema et al,[15] 2008 N = 28	NT-pro-BNP	MAS showed improvement	Only MAS improved NT-pro-BNP	N/A Parallel study
Gagnadoux et al,[14] 2009 N = 69	PSG Nottinham QoL Osler test	MAS and CPAP improved AHI Improvement Improvement	CPAP>MAS MAS = CPAP MAS = CPAP	71.2% MAS 8.5% CPAP 14.5% MAS = CPAP
Trzepizur et al,[20] 2009 N = 12	Microvascular reactivity PSG Blood pressure	MAS and CPAP Improvement AHI and ODI No difference	MAS = CPAP MAS = CPAP MAS = CPAP	Not described
Aarab et al,[19] 2011 N = 57	PSG ESS	Improvement AHI Improvement	MAS = CPAP MAS = CPAP	N/A Parallel study
Aarab et al,[2] 2011 N = 43	PSG after 1 y ESS	Stable AHI improvement Additional sleepiness improvement	CPAP>MAS MAS = CPAP	N/A Parallel study
Holley et al,[21] 2011 N = 378	PSG	Improved AHI	MAS = CPAP for mild to moderate CPAP>MAS severe OSA	Not described

Abbreviations: ESS, Epworth Sleepiness Scale; NT-pro-BNP, concentration of the amino-terminal fragment of pro- brain natriuretic peptide; ODI, oxygen desaturation index; PSG, polysomnogram.

one type of therapy for patients with OSA who are potentially good candidates for MAS therapy.

Titration

Analogous to the pressure of a CPAP mask, the amount of mandibular advancement produced by a MAD that will effectively reduce the number of apneas will vary from patient to patient. The amount of pressure required for each patient cannot be predetermined based on OSA severity or craniofacial characteristics; as such the magnitude of advancement needs to be determined through a titration procedure. Typically, the amount of advancement is initially set at 66% of maximum protrusion, and over a period of weeks, patients slowly increase the advancement by adjusting the appliance until there is resolution of subjective OSA symptoms. At this point, a follow-up polysomnogram (PSG) with the device worn is required to ensure adequate improvement to breathing during sleep. A schematic of the treatment protocol can be seen in **Fig. 1**.

Additional advancement of the appliance by titration carried out during this follow-up PSG has been shown to further increase the success rate of OA therapy.[30,31] This advancement is achieved by simply having the sleep technologist wake and ask the patient to increase the protrusion of the appliance should there be persistent snoring or events related to adverse breathing. Several studies have evaluated whether a titration of mandibular advancement during polysomnography could be used as a predictor and accelerate MAS treatment, similar to CPAP titration.[30,32–35] These studies had mixed results in predicting the amount of mandibular advancement needed for successful MAS therapy, and overnight titration of MAS at appliance delivery remains an experimental approach.

The importance of titration to enhance the efficacy of MAS therapy is highlighted by a closer examination of randomized controlled trials (see **Table 1**) comparing CPAP to MAS. Most of these studies have found that MAS and CPAP have a similar impact on daytime sleepiness and quality of life.[2,3,12–15,17,18,35] In 2 other studies, Engleman[11] and Lam[16] have reported an inferiority of MAS compared with CPAP; however, it is important to note that fixed, nontitratable, single-jaw position appliances were used for their patients. Previous reports on effective single-jaw positioners have proposed that, if this type of appliance is used, there should be the opportunity to remake these devices with further mandibular advancement, which represents titration with multiple appliances.[36] Also, the increased likelihood of providing successful therapy with adjustable compared with fixed appliances is especially evident in cases of moderate and severe OSA.[37] It is clear in the literature that customizing the fit of the MAS, with the use of a custom-made appliance to the patient's specific oral anatomy, and determining the ideal anterior position of the mandible via titration of the amount of advancement are crucial to optimizing the effectiveness of therapy.

APPLIANCE DESIGN

There are a multitude of MAS designs with various methods of adjustment and retention mechanisms available on the marketplace today. As such it is easy to imagine these differences contributing to some of the variability observed in the results of clinical studies investigating MAS effectiveness. The possible influence of various MAS design features on the management of subjective symptoms during OSA treatment was recently examined in a systematic review.[38] The results suggest that an appliance with titratable mandibular advancement that is found acceptable by patients because of greater comfort and retention, and being custom made (not prefabricated), will be

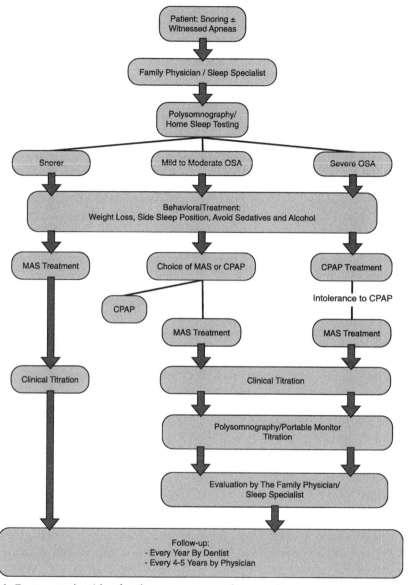

Fig. 1. Treatment algorithm for the management of OSA with an oral appliance.

successful at improving sleep-disordered breathing signs and symptoms. It is also noted that the optimum amount of advancement might not necessarily be the maximum achievable forward position of the mandible. The investigators also reported that the amount of vertical opening did not impact significantly on the appliance design. Isono and collaborators[39] found that an increase in jaw opening would decrease the upper airway area. Pitsis and colleagues[40] found that a 10-mm increase in the jaw opening did not make significant differences in the AHI, but a highest percentage of patients developed temporomandibular joint symptoms with the greater jaw opening. More recently Nikolopoulou and collaborators[41] evaluated an increase in vertical dimensions without mandibular advancement. They concluded that without mandibular protrusion an increase in vertical dimension was associated with an aggravation of OSA. In summary, there is no preferred MAD design, as long as it is properly custom made for the patient, patient comfort is achieved, it has good retention, and most importantly allows for mandibular advancement and titration to optimize treatment outcome.

MAS EFFECTS ON SLEEPINESS AND QUALITY OF LIFE

MAS have been shown to be effective in improving subjective and objective daytime sleepiness in patients with OSAS when compared with placebo and improves sleepiness to the same degree as the CPAP.[23,42] Aarab and colleagues[2] examined the effects of MAS and CPAP treatment 12 months following initial titration for patients with mild to moderate OSA. They found that CPAP reduced AHI slightly better than MAS and that the improvements in AHI were stable over the 12-month time period; however, subjective sleepiness progressively improved for all patients in the same time frame. They concluded that a lack of long-term differences in improvements in sleepiness between the MAS and the CPAP groups may indicate that the larger improvements in AHI values in the CPAP group are not clinically relevant. Johal and collaborators[42] found that MAS therapy significantly improved the energy/vitality domain of quality of life and reduced subjective sleepiness in a group of patients with OSA preselected for a favorable treatment outcome using sleep nasendoscopy. Similar improvements were not seen in a conservatively managed group. There were some interesting findings in a study from Gagnadoux and colleagues[14] whereby MAS showed a greater improvement compared with CPAP in a variety of profiles of quality of life (Nottingham Health Profile), such as physical mobility, social isolation, pain, emotional function, and sleep. MAS treatment may not improve AHI as much as CPAP, but consistently throughout various studies, does significantly improve their quality of life. For patients to adhere to treatment, it is crucial that patients feel better and acknowledge the importance of treatment.

MAS INFLUENCE ON LONG-TERM HEALTH EFFECTS OF OSA

OSA is considered a risk factor for cardiovascular disease, including systemic hypertension, congestive heart failure, arrhythmias, and stroke[43]; and recent studies have demonstrated a significant increased risk of fatal cardiovascular events in patients with untreated sleep apnea.[44] There is currently initial evidence demonstrating that MAS therapy can play a role in reducing the risk of these adverse health effects associated with OSA.

MAS treatment has been shown to reduce systemic blood pressure in several studies, including 2 randomized controlled trials with intention-to-treat analysis[3,45] and 3 nonrandomized prospective studies.[46–48] Compared with a placebo, the management of OSA with MAS can significantly reduce systolic and diastolic pressure, while lowering the mean blood pressure measurements by 3.6 mm Hg.[45] Barnes and colleagues[3] examined nocturnal blood pressure levels and demonstrated no change in blood pressure with CPAP treatment, whereas MAS treatment significantly improved the nocturnal diastolic blood pressure and increased the proportion of patients with a normal nighttime dip in blood pressure. Improvements in blood pressure levels have been observed to persist for at least 3 years with continued MAS therapy.[48] A correlation between the improvement in AHI and decrease in blood pressure after MAS treatment has also been found.[46]

In an examination of biomarkers of oxidative stress and inflammation, the endothelial function in a MAS treatment group normalized compared with a reference non-OSA group of patients.[24] Interestingly these changes were observable after 12 months of treatment despite residual sleep-disordered breathing (average AHI of 19 per hour). Treatment effects of MAS have also been found on the autonomic nervous system with improvements in cardiovascular variability.[49]

PREDICTORS OF MAS TREATMENT SUCCESS

There are various studies on the prediction of MAS treatment success. Treatment success may be inversely related to pretreatment severity, but this relationship may be a function of the definition of treatment success, although one study has shown that the higher AHI pretreatment, the greater decrease in AHI could be achieved.[35] In an evaluation of the literature, there is a common agreement that MAS is likely to be more effective in patients that are younger[50,51]; have a lower body mass index[14,51]; have a smaller neck circumference[8]; and have positional OSA,[36,50,52] whereby patients have a higher number of respiratory events in the supine compared with the lateral sleep position. Women also have shown a higher percentage of success.[36] Despite these findings, further prospective studies are required to better predict which patients will experience a greater level of success through OA therapy.

SIDE EFFECTS OF MAS

Although effective and well tolerated, MAS have known side effects, including dry mouth, increase in salivation, dental discomfort, transitory temporomandibular dysfunction, and most commonly, unwanted dental movement. Previous studies have shown a significant decrease in overbite (OB) and overjet (OJ) after long-term appliance use.[53–55] Martinez and colleagues[53] found a mean OB reduction of 0.81 mm and OJ reduction of 1.1 mm from 15 patients with OSA with 4.8 years of MAS use. Similarly, Marklund[54] found reduction of both OB and OJ by 0.6 mm from a 5-year follow-up of 155 patients with OSA. In the longest follow-up period published to date, Almeida and colleagues[55] demonstrated that the use of an adjustable MAD for a mean period of 7.3 years has a significant impact on the occlusion, with a mean reduction of 1.9 mm and 1.2 mm for OB and OJ respectively. In that study, many changes were described as favorable changes to the patient's occlusion, as seen in **Fig. 2**. It is important to emphasize that these changes are mainly related to dentoalveolar

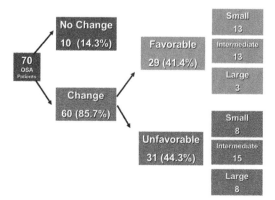

Fig. 2. The occlusal changes in 70 patients after an average of 7.4 years of MAS use.

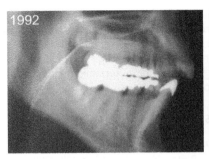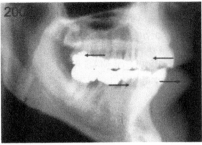

- Retroclination of the maxillary incisors
- Distal tipping of the maxillary molars
- Proclination of the mandibular incisors
- Mesial tipping of the mandibular molars
- NO Changes in condyle position

Fig. 3. Dentoalveolar changes after 9 years of MAS use.

changes and not condylar remodeling (**Fig. 3**). Because MAS are a life-long treatment and changes do continue overtime, it is crucial to advise patients before initiation of treatment that some type of occlusion changes are likely to happen, and the dentist should ideally collect cephalometric radiographs, dental models, and intraoral photographs over the course of the treatment. MAS are an important treatment option for OSA, which is a life-threatening disease that requires long-term treatment. Changes in the occlusion should not stop patients from using MAS, unless patients are willing to start using CPAP. If patients are willing to use CPAP, they should be advised not to use the nasal masks because these also change the occlusion.[56]

ORAL APPLIANCES FOR THE TREATMENT OF SLEEP-DISORDERED BREATHING IN CHILDREN AND ADOLESCENTS

The use of MAS, which can be highly effective in the treatment of adult OSA, has more limited applications in younger patients. In a growing child or adolescent, such an appliance can result in dramatic skeletal and dentoalveolar changes, as observed with the use of functional orthodontic appliances. Such concerns over bite alterations preclude widespread use. However, in class II retrognathic patients, these occlusal changes are favorable, and functional appliance treatment has been proposed as a means to treat retrognathic children suffering from sleep-disordered breathing. In a randomized controlled study of 7-year-old children suffering from OSA, Villa and colleagues[57] observed a mean reduction in AHI of 7.1 ± 4.6 to 2.6 ± 2.2, whereas no reduction in AHI was seen in the control group. Similar positive outcomes were demonstrated in an older cohort of retrognathic adolescents with sleep-disordered breathing in the absence of tonsillar hypertrophy, where Schutz and colleagues[58] effectively normalized the respiratory disturbance index with orthopedic correction of mandibular deficiency.

An equally common appliance in orthodontic treatment, the use of a rapid maxillary expander has been shown to be effective in reducing sleep respiratory disturbances in patients with[59] and without[60] tonsillar hypertrophy. Furthermore, these results have been shown to remain up to 36 months following the expansion protocol.[61] However, the greatest utility of this protocol may be as an adjunctive therapy for children who have incomplete resolution of their symptoms following the removal of enlarged tonsils and adenoids. Guilleminault and colleagues[62] compared adenotonsillectomy surgery with palatal expansion in a crossover study design of young children diagnosed with OSA by PSG. In their sample of 31 children who had tonsillar hypertrophy and a narrow and high palate, an equal level of improvement to AHI and reported symptoms was found after treatment with either intervention; however, both the surgical and orthodontic treatments were required for complete resolution of symptoms and normalization of AHI, which occurred in 29 of the 31 children.

There is emerging evidence that treatment with oral appliances for maxillary expansion or mandibular advancement can be an effective therapy in children suffering from sleep-disordered breathing, particularly if a craniofacial discrepancy plays a significantly role in the patient's disease. However, further research is needed to elicit in which patients this treatment will be most effective and when such treatment can act as an adjunct or as the first line of therapy for children and adolescents with sleep-disordered breathing.

REFERENCES

1. Kushida CA, Morgenthaler TI, Littner MR, et al. Practice parameters for the treatment of snoring and obstructive sleep apnea with oral appliances: an update for 2005. Sleep 2006;29(2):240–3.
2. Aarab G, Lobbezoo F, Heymans MW, et al. Long-term follow-up of a randomized controlled trial of oral appliance therapy in obstructive sleep apnea. Respiration 2011;82(2):162–8.
3. Barnes M, McEvoy RD, Banks S, et al. Efficacy of positive airway pressure and oral appliance in mild to moderate obstructive sleep apnea. Am J Respir Crit Care Med 2004;170(6):656–64.
4. Blanco J, Zamarrón C, Abeleira Pazos MT, et al. Prospective evaluation of an oral appliance in the treatment of obstructive sleep apnea syndrome. Sleep Breath 2005;9(1):20–5.
5. Gotsopoulos H, Chen C, Qian J, et al. Oral appliance therapy improves symptoms in obstructive sleep apnea: a randomized, controlled trial. Am J Respir Crit Care Med 2002;166(5):743–8.
6. Hans MG, Nelson S, Luks VG, et al. Comparison of two dental devices for treatment of obstructive sleep apnea syndrome (OSAS). Am J Orthod Dentofacial Orthop 1997;111(5):562–70.
7. Johnston CD, Gleadhill IC, Cinnamond MJ, et al. Mandibular advancement appliances and obstructive sleep apnoea: a randomized clinical trial. Eur J Orthod 2002;24(3):251–62.
8. Mehta A, Qian J, Petocz P, et al. A randomized, controlled study of a mandibular advancement splint for obstructive sleep apnea. Am J Respir Crit Care Med 2001;163(6):1457–61.
9. Naismith SL, Winter VR, Hickie IB, et al. Effect of oral appliance therapy on neurobehavioral functioning in obstructive sleep apnea: a randomized controlled trial. J Clin Sleep Med 2005;1(4):374–80.
10. Petri N, Svanholt P, Solow B, et al. Mandibular advancement appliance for obstructive sleep apnoea: results of a randomised placebo controlled trial using parallel group design. J Sleep Res 2008;17(2):221–9.
11. Engleman HM, McDonald JP, Graham D, et al. Randomized crossover trial of two treatments for sleep apnea/hypopnea syndrome: continuous positive airway pressure and mandibular repositioning splint. Am J Respir Crit Care Med 2002;166(6):855–9.

12. Ferguson KA, Ono T, Lowe AA, et al. A randomized crossover study of an oral appliance vs nasal-continuous positive airway pressure in the treatment of mild-moderate obstructive sleep apnea. Chest 1996;109(5):1269–75.

13. Ferguson KA, Ono T, Lowe AA, et al. A short-term controlled trial of an adjustable oral appliance for the treatment of mild to moderate obstructive sleep apnoea. Thorax 1997;52(4):362–8.

14. Gagnadoux F, Fleury B, Vielle B, et al. Titrated mandibular advancement versus positive airway pressure for sleep apnoea. Eur Respir J 2009;34(4): 914–20.

15. Hoekema A, Voors AA, Wijkstra PJ, et al. Effects of oral appliances and CPAP on the left ventricle and natriuretic peptides. Int J Cardiol 2008;128(2):232–9.

16. Lam B, Sam K, Mok WY, et al. Randomised study of three non-surgical treatments in mild to moderate obstructive sleep apnoea. Thorax 2007;62(4):354–9.

17. Randerath WJ, Heise M, Hinz R, et al. An individually adjustable oral appliance vs continuous positive airway pressure in mild-to-moderate obstructive sleep apnea syndrome. Chest 2002;122(2):569–75.

18. Tan YK, L'Estrange PR, Luo YM, et al. Mandibular advancement splints and continuous positive airway pressure in patients with obstructive sleep apnoea: a randomized cross-over trial. Eur J Orthod 2002;24(3):239–49.

19. Aarab G, Lobbezoo F, Hamburger HL, et al. Oral appliance therapy versus nasal continuous positive airway pressure in obstructive sleep apnea: a randomized, placebo-controlled trial. Respiration 2011;81(5):411–9.

20. Trzepizur W, Gagnadoux F, Abraham P, et al. Microvascular endothelial function in obstructive sleep apnea: impact of continuous positive airway pressure and mandibular advancement. Sleep Med 2009;10(7):746–52.

21. Holley AB, Lettieri CJ, Shah AA. Efficacy of an adjustable oral appliance and comparison with continuous positive airway pressure for the treatment of obstructive sleep apnea syndrome. Chest 2011;140(6):1511–6.

22. Hoekema A, Stegenga B, Bakker M, et al. Simulated driving in obstructive sleep apnoea-hypopnoea; effects of oral appliances and continuous positive airway pressure. Sleep Breath 2007;11(3):129–38.

23. Lim J, Lasserson TJ, Fleetham J, et al. Oral appliances for obstructive sleep apnoea. Cochrane Database Syst Rev 2006;1:CD004435.

24. Itzhaki S, Dorchin H, Clark G, et al. The effects of 1-year treatment with a herbst mandibular advancement splint on obstructive sleep apnea, oxidative stress, and endothelial function. Chest 2007;131(3):740–9.

25. Chan ASL, Sutherland K, Schwab RJ, et al. The effect of mandibular advancement on upper airway structure in obstructive sleep apnoea. Thorax 2010;65(8): 726–32.

26. McTaggart-Cowan HM, Marra CA, Yang Y, et al. The validity of generic and condition-specific preference-based instruments: the ability to discriminate asthma control status. Qual Life Res 2008;17(3):453–62.

27. Vanderveken OM, Devolder A, Marklund M, et al. Comparison of a custom-made and a thermoplastic oral appliance for the treatment of mild sleep apnea. Am J Respir Crit Care Med 2008;178(2):197–202.

28. Friedman M, Pulver T, Wilson MN, et al. Otolaryngology office-based treatment of obstructive sleep apnea-hypopnea syndrome with titratable and nontitratable thermoplastic mandibular advancement devices. Otolaryngol Head Neck Surg 2010;143(1):78–84.

29. Lowe AA, Sjöholm TT, Ryan CF, et al. Treatment, airway and compliance effects of a titratable oral appliance. Sleep 2000;23(Suppl 4):S172–8.

30. Krishnan V, Collop NA, Scherr SC. An evaluation of a titration strategy for prescription of oral appliances for obstructive sleep apnea. Chest 2008;133(5): 1135–41.
31. Almeida FR, Parker JA, Hodges JS, et al. Effect of a titration polysomnogram on treatment success with a mandibular repositioning appliance. J Clin Sleep Med 2009;5(3):198–204.
32. Raphaelson MA, Alpher EJ, Bakker KW, et al. Oral appliance therapy for obstructive sleep apnea syndrome: progressive mandibular advancement during polysomnography. Cranio 1998;16(1):44–50.
33. Pételle B, Vincent G, Gagnadoux F, et al. One-night mandibular advancement titration for obstructive sleep apnea syndrome: a pilot study. Am J Respir Crit Care Med 2002;165(8):1150–3.
34. Tsai WH, Vazquez JC, Oshima T, et al. Remotely controlled mandibular positioner predicts efficacy of oral appliances in sleep apnea. Am J Respir Crit Care Med 2004;170(4):366–70.
35. Kuna ST, Giarraputo PC, Stanton DC, et al. Evaluation of an oral mandibular advancement titration appliance. Oral Surg Oral Med Oral Pathol Oral Radiol Endod 2006;101(5):593–603.
36. Marklund M, Stenlund H, Franklin KA. Mandibular advancement devices in 630 men and women with obstructive sleep apnea and snoring: tolerability and predictors of treatment success. Chest 2004;125(4):1270–8.
37. Lettieri CJ, Paolino N, Eliasson AH, et al. Comparison of adjustable and fixed oral appliances for the treatment of obstructive sleep apnea. J Clin Sleep Med 2011; 7(5):439–45.
38. Ahrens A, McGrath C, Hägg U. Subjective efficacy of oral appliance design features in the management of obstructive sleep apnea: a systematic review. Am J Orthod Dentofacial Orthop 2010;138(5):559–76.
39. Isono S. Influences of head positions and bite opening on collapsibility of the passive pharynx. J Appl Physiol 2004;97(1):339–46.
40. Pitsis AJ, Darendeliler MA, Gotsopoulos H, et al. Effect of vertical dimension on efficacy of oral appliance therapy in obstructive sleep apnea. Am J Respir Crit Care Med 2002;166(6):860–4.
41. Nikolopoulou M, Naeije M, Aarab G, et al. The effect of raising the bite without mandibular protrusion on obstructive sleep apnoea. J Oral Rehabil 2011;38(9):643–7.
42. Johal A, Battagel J, Hector M. Controlled, prospective trial of psychosocial function before and after mandibular advancement splint therapy. Am J Orthod Dentofacial Orthop 2011;139(5):581–7.
43. Bradley TD, Floras JS. Obstructive sleep apnoea and its cardiovascular consequences. Lancet 2009;373(9657):82–93.
44. Marin J, Carrizo S, Vicente E, et al. Long-term cardiovascular outcomes in men with obstructive sleep apnoea-hypopnoea with or without treatment with continuous positive airway pressure: an observational study. Lancet 2005;365(9464): 1046–53.
45. Gotsopoulos H, Kelly JJ, Cistulli PA. Oral appliance therapy reduces blood pressure in obstructive sleep apnea: a randomized, controlled trial. Sleep 2004;27(5): 934–41.
46. Yoshida K. Effect on blood pressure of oral appliance therapy for sleep apnea syndrome. Int J Prosthodont 2006;19(1):61–6.
47. Otsuka R, de Almeida FR, Lowe AA, et al. The effect of oral appliance therapy on blood pressure in patients with obstructive sleep apnea. Sleep Breath 2006; 10(1):29–36.

48. Andrén A, Sjöquist M, Tegelberg A. Effects on blood pressure after treatment of obstructive sleep apnoea with a mandibular advancement appliance - a three-year follow-up. J Oral Rehabil 2009;36(10):719–25.

49. Coruzzi P, Gualerzi M, Bernkopf E, et al. Autonomic cardiac modulation in obstructive sleep apnea: effect of an oral jaw-positioning appliance. Chest 2006;130(5):1362–8.

50. Liu Y, Park YC, Lowe AA, et al. Supine cephalometric analyses of an adjustable oral appliance used in the treatment of obstructive sleep apnea. Sleep Breath 2000;4(2):59–66.

51. Liu Y, Lowe AA, Fleetham JA, et al. Cephalometric and physiologic predictors of the efficacy of an adjustable oral appliance for treating obstructive sleep apnea. Am J Orthod Dentofacial Orthop 2001;120(6):639–47.

52. Yoshida K. Influence of sleep posture on response to oral appliance therapy for sleep apnea syndrome. Sleep 2001;24(5):538–44.

53. Martínez-Gomis J, Willaert E, Nogues L, et al. Five years of sleep apnea treatment with a mandibular advancement device. Side effects and technical complications. Angle Orthod 2010;80(1):30–6.

54. Marklund M. Predictors of long-term orthodontic side effects from mandibular advancement devices in patients with snoring and obstructive sleep apnea. Am J Orthod Dentofacial Orthop 2006;129(2):214–21.

55. Almeida de FR, Lowe AA, Otsuka R, et al. Long-term sequellae of oral appliance therapy in obstructive sleep apnea patients: part 2. Study-model analysis. Am J Orthod Dentofacial Orthop 2006;129(2):205–13.

56. Tsuda H, Almeida FR, Tsuda T, et al. Craniofacial changes after 2 years of nasal continuous positive airway pressure use in patients with obstructive sleep apnea. Chest 2010;138(4):870–4.

57. Villa M, Bernkopf E, Pagani J. Randomized controlled study of an oral jaw-positioning appliance for the treatment of obstructive sleep apnea in children with malocclusion. Am J Respir Crit Care Med 2002;165(1):123–7.

58. Schütz TC, Dominguez GC, Hallinan MP, et al. Class II correction improves nocturnal breathing in adolescents. Angle Orthod 2011;81(2):222–8.

59. Villa MP, Malagola C, Pagani J, et al. Rapid maxillary expansion in children with obstructive sleep apnea syndrome: 12-month follow-up. Sleep Med 2007;8(2):128–34.

60. Pirelli P, Saponara M, de Rosa C, et al. Orthodontics and obstructive sleep apnea in children. Med Clin North Am 2010;94(3):517–29.

61. Villa MP, Rizzoli A, Miano S, et al. Efficacy of rapid maxillary expansion in children with obstructive sleep apnea syndrome: 36 months of follow-up. Sleep Breath 2011;15(2):179–84.

62. Guilleminault C, Monteyrol PJ, Huynh NT, et al. Adeno-tonsillectomy and rapid maxillary distraction in pre-pubertal children, a pilot study. Sleep Breath 2011;15(2):173–7.

Use of Portable Monitoring for Sleep-Disordered Breathing Treated with an Oral Appliance

Dennis R. Bailey, DDS[a,b],*

KEYWORDS

- Oral appliances • Portable monitoring • Home sleep study
- Screening • Titration

The potential use of a portable monitor to assess the outcome of treatment with an oral appliance would ideally be performed by the dentist who is managing the patient's sleep-disordered breathing. A sleep medicine physician or sleep center may also perform such a study. The dentist may be using portable monitoring as a means of assessing the response to the oral appliance after an initial titration period along with assessment of the patient's symptom resolution before referral back to the patient's physician, sleep medicine specialist, or for a follow-up polysomnogram. Portable monitoring may be one of the most cost-effective ways for the treating dentist to assess the outcome or effect of the oral appliance, to determine if further adjustment/modification to the appliance is needed, and to retest to determine the current status following any adjustment or modification.

This article emphasizes the use of portable monitors primarily for follow-up care and assessment as opposed to diagnosis or, as it is sometimes referred to, screening. Many have advocated the use of portable monitor type devices as a means by which the dentist can screen patients who might be at risk for sleep apnea.[1,2] This is clearly a diagnostic procedure for a potential medical condition that is not within the scope of dental practice at this time. Portable monitors, specifically level 3 devices, have limited use as an alternative to the overnight polysomnogram (level 1) as an effective instrument for the diagnosis of sleep apnea.[3]

This article originally appeared in *Sleep Medicine Clinics, Volume 6, Number 3, 2011.*
[a] Orofacial Pain and Dental Sleep Medicine Department, UCLA School of Dentistry, Los Angeles, CA, USA
[b] Dental Sleep Mini-Residency, UCLA School of Dentistry, Los Angeles, CA, USA
* 8400 East Prentice Avenue, Suite 804, Greenwood Village, CO 80111.
E-mail address: RMC4E@aol.com

HISTORY AND CURRENT STATUS: A CASE REPORT

A 54-year old man presents to a dentist who has advanced training and is competent in dental sleep medicine and the use of oral appliances for managing sleep-disordered breathing. He was referred to the dentist by the sleep center where the polysomnogram was done and his primary care physician, mainly because he was unable to tolerate continuous positive airway pressure (CPAP) despite trying numerous masks. He had a consultation with an otolaryngologist about possible surgery and was also informed that an oral appliance would be more appropriate at this time. His Epworth Sleepiness Scale score was 13 (the normal value is >10) and the apnea/hypopnea index (AHI) was 21 per hour of sleep. His body mass index is 28 kg/m^2 and his neck size is 40 cm. He has been diagnosed with hypertension, which is controlled with Lisinopril and hydrochlorothiazide. With medication, his blood pressure is 121/82. He denies having any other health-related issues, specifically cardio-vascular disease or diabetes. He reports that his sleep onset is within 15 minutes but his sleep is restless with multiple awakenings (2–3 per night) and he gets 6 hours of sleep a night on average. He reports that he has snored for more than 20 years; and in the last 5 years the snoring has become more problematic and observed apnea has occurred.

A formal orofacial and airway evaluation was performed as has been described and recommended for the dentist who performs this type of service.[4] This also included an evaluation of the nasal airway. During the evaluation, he denied being a mouth breather at night and has no difficulty breathing through the nose. However, nasal dilation (commonly known as the Cottle test) improved the patient's ability to nose breath. He did report trying nasal strips for nasal dilation but they were not effective for the snoring and did not seem to affect his sleep.

By virtue of testing, it was determined that with the mandible repositioned, which included opening the vertical approximately 5 mm and advancing the mandible 2–3 mm, he believed his airway was improved and he would not snore. At this point, an oral appliance was determined to be an appropriate treatment and the necessary records were obtained for the fabrication of the oral appliance.

At the first follow-up 2 weeks after receiving the oral appliance, he reports that the snoring is significantly improved, he feels his sleep and feeling of being tired and sleepy during the day are improved. He also feels he is more productive at work and not as tired at the end of the day. Some adjustment to the oral appliance is done mainly for comfort and he is reappointed in a month. He has had the oral appliance for 6 weeks and reports that his symptoms continue to improve and his snoring is present but much improved. Because of the snoring, his mandible is advanced approximately 2 mm and with this change he feels his breathing is also improved. He is reappointed for a follow-up visit in another month.

At the third follow-up visit he reports that the snoring is no longer present according to his wife and he continues to believe that he has improved energy levels and is sleeping through the night. He awakens rested and wakes up without an alarm most mornings. By report, his initial complaints and neurocognitive symptoms are improved (**Table 1**). At this point no further adjustment is deemed necessary and he is reappointed for a follow-up visit in 2 months.

He has now had the oral appliance for more than 4 months and is satisfied with the results. At this time a portable monitoring sleep study to assess the effect of the oral appliance and to determine if any further adjustment is needed, is arranged. It is explained that this is not the same type of sleep study that he had initially. This study is not for diagnosis of sleep apnea (this has already been done) but to determine if the

Table 1
Case report: symptoms of obstructive sleep apnea before and after use of an oral appliance

Symptom	Before Oral Appliance Use	With Oral Appliance Use
Snoring	Present	Resolved
Epworth Sleepiness Scale score	13	5
Excessive daytime sleepiness	Present	Reduced/improved
Drowsy driving	Present	Eliminated
Concentration	Difficult	Improved
Energy levels	Low	Improved/resolved
Observed apnea	Present at times	None
Mood swings/irritable	Present	Resolved
Restless sleep	Present	Resolved
Awakenings each night	2 to 3	None now
Headaches	Occasional (2–3 a week)	None

appliance is managing the apnea adequately. The appropriate consent forms are completed and he is scheduled to have the study done.

The portable monitoring study is completed after the patient is instructed on the use and application of the equipment. He will do a 1-night study and return the equipment to the office the next day. At that time, the data will be downloaded for review. The results of the portable monitoring study reveal that the AHI is now 7 and his blood oxygen levels are in the 90% or greater range, nearly 100% of the time. His Epworth Sleepiness Scale score is now 5. At this time he seems to be deriving a reasonable outcome with the oral appliance. A report is generated and will be sent to the referring physician, to the sleep center where the initial sleep study was performed, and to any other physicians who are directly involved with the patient's care. A decision will be made regarding the need for an attended level 1 sleep study to further substantiate the effect of the oral appliance and his current level of apnea.

Portable Monitoring for Diagnosis Before Oral Appliance Therapy

The dental sleep medicine practitioner is the one who will most likely be providing an oral appliance. However, the use of portable monitoring to screen for sleep-disordered breathing in those patients who may be at risk for sleep apnea is not within the scope of practice by the dentist. Despite the advanced training the dentist may have in sleep medicine, they, like most primary care physicians, are not well-versed in the recognition of coexisting sleep disorders that may present as the same type of symptoms as sleep-disordered breathing.[5] Even with advanced training, the level 3 portable monitor will not provide adequate information to allow for the diagnosis of comorbid sleep disorders such as central sleep apnea, periodic limb movements (PLMs), parasomnias, various circadian rhythm sleep disorders, or narcolepsy. In addition, the portable monitor is not indicated for use as a general screening device in an asymptomatic population. The more appropriate action is to identify those patients who are at risk for sleep-disordered breathing. Once it is established that the patient is at risk, the patient should be referred to their primary care physician or to a sleep center for a polysomnogram.

In general, the use of the level 3 portable monitor is not accepted as the optimal method for diagnosing sleep-disordered breathing at the present time. The gold standard continues to be the overnight polysomnogram.[3] However, there are numerous articles that support the use of these portable monitors for patients with high pretest probability of being at risk for sleep-disordered breathing.[6,7]

The main issue is that the sensitivity and specificity of these devices at an AHI less than 15 is not as good compared with an AHI greater than 15. One study did find that portable monitoring was most reliable at an AHI of 10 or more.[8] In addition, portable monitors may actually underestimate the severity of sleep apnea. This is related to the computation of the AHI and more specifically, the respiratory disturbance index (RDI) per hour of recording time because of the difference in total sleep time versus total recording time.[9]

Another issue related to diagnosis using a portable monitor, even if it is being used to assess just snoring, is if the outcome is negative (RDI >5), then the patient may not seek or obtain treatment. Who then assumes the liability for the medical consequences of the sleep apnea? Given that the portable monitor may underestimate the degree of sleep apnea, this is of particular concern in patients who are asymptomatic and may only perceive the issue as snoring, not sleep apnea.

The role of the dentist, regardless of the level of training, is to perform risk assessment for a sleep-disordered breathing condition. Risk assessment is initially done by having an awareness of the following[4]:

1. Assessment of findings through questions in the health history (screening)
2. Assessment of the most common symptoms of sleep-disordered breathing
3. Awareness of existing medical conditions that indicate the possible risk for sleep-disordered breathing
4. Use of standard questionnaires such as the Epworth Sleepiness Scale or the Berlin questionnaire
5. Findings from the head/oral/airway clinical evaluation.

Based on the assessment of risk and comorbid conditions, the patient is referred to a sleep medicine specialist or for a sleep study. That study would most likely be a polysomnogram.

Portable Monitoring for Progressive/Follow-Up Testing with Oral Appliance Therapy

The use of level 3 portable monitoring based on published clinical guidelines has been recommended (consensus) for the purpose of determining the effectiveness of oral appliance therapy for sleep-disordered breathing.[3] This is stated as follows:

> Sect 1.4 PM: "Portable Monitoring (PM) may be indicted to monitor the response to non-CPAP treatments for obstructive sleep apnea, including oral appliances, upper airway surgery, and weight loss."

Furthermore, the use of level 3 portable monitors for assessment of the effectiveness of an oral appliance after the final adjustment is a practice parameter guideline.[10] A more practical point of view would potentially use the portable monitor at various points in the titration process of the treatment to determine if added adjustment or modification is needed before a more definitive sleep study. Assuming that the level 3 portable monitor is reliable, its use would contribute to improvement in consistent and successful use of the oral appliance for the management of sleep apnea.[8] In some cases, the level 3 portable monitoring study may actually be satisfactory in determining that the oral appliance is adequately addressing the sleep-disordered breathing. This is a decision that ultimately should be made by the sleep medicine specialist, not the treating dentist.

The American Academy of Dental Sleep Medicine (AADSM) in 2005 also established a position as it relates to the use of portable monitoring.[11] The position that has been taken is that the use of portable monitoring should be restricted to use for titration of the oral appliance (the need for adjustment and modification) for an enhanced effect and to document the effectiveness of the treatment. Furthermore, the use of portable monitors "as a screening tool" designed to identify those patients who may require an overnight polysomnogram is not endorsed at this time. In 2009, the AADSM published a treatment protocol for oral appliances that indicated that portable monitoring was applicable for gathering objective data for the purpose of oral appliance titration.[12]

Based on studies that have looked at the use of level 3 portable monitors compared with polysomnograms for diagnosis, it seems that the portable monitor should provide information to determine that the oral appliance is adequately resolving the sleep-disordered breathing and has also improved the patient's symptoms. Concern for the recognition of other coexisting sleep disorders is not an issue with the use of this technology because these conditions have most likely been recognized (diagnosed) from the original polysomnogram and their management is being considered aside from the use of the oral appliance for the sleep-disordered breathing. Consequently, not all of the parameters of the sleep study are needed to ascertain that the oral appliance is effectively managing the sleep-disordered breathing. The parameters of greatest value in evaluating the effectiveness of the oral appliance are listed in **Table 2**.

Assessment of the AHI based on the use of a thermistor may underestimate the number of hypopneas.[13] Measurement of nasal pressure is more sensitive but may be subject to signal loss. More importantly, mouth breathing will also decrease the effectiveness of this measuring device. The presence of mouth breathing in patients with sleep apnea is a significant issue that is often underevaluated and insufficiently addressed. Before any testing using the portable monitor, an effort should be made to address mouth breathing when using an oral appliance and strategies should be used to improve the nasal airway and nasal breathing while using the appliance. This is best done using nasal rinses, nasal dilation, and in some cases, nasal airway surgery. Myofunctional tongue therapy has also been shown to be helpful with improvement of the tongue posture and by achieving a lip seal, which may improve nasal breathing during sleep.[14] If the patient continues to be predominately a mouth breather, this needs to be considered when the level 3 portable monitor is being

Table 2 Parameters of value to determine effectiveness of an oral appliance with portable monitoring	
Parameter Being Tested	**Significance**
AHI	Needs to be less than 10 and ideally less than 5 (not always possible due to sensitivity and specificity for ≤ 10 or ≤ 15) based on the device
Snoring	Need to evaluate presence or resolution If present, for what period of time
Oxygen saturation	Ideally needs to be in the 90% range nearly 100% of the time Need to distinguish parameter of desaturation (3% vs 4%)
Sleep position	Not always available on all devices
Sleep bruxism (optional)	Ideal from the standpoint of the dentist and as a coexisting condition Not available on portable monitors; can be adapted on selected devices

used for titration. In this type of situation, the oral appliance should be titrated to an optimum outcome and the patient should have an overnight polysomnogram to better ascertain the effectiveness of the oral appliance.

A poster presentation at the AADSM annual meeting in June 2010 addressed the use of portable monitoring (home sleep monitoring) for the purpose of guiding the titration of the oral appliance. The study looked at 32 subjects who had been diagnosed with moderate to severe sleep apnea. The testing device reported the AHI, the amount of time that the oxygen saturation was less than 90% and the O_2 nadir.[15] By using such a system it was determined that the oral appliance was effective in 71% of the patients. It was also found that the O_2 nadir increased by 4.5% and the percent of time the oxygen saturation was less than 90% improved by 64%. This was also correlated to the patient's symptoms; there was a significant improvement in quality of life and daytime sleepiness was improved in 90% of the patients in the study. The conclusion here is that once the patient has experienced a subjective improvement in the initial symptoms, the portable monitor can be used to determine if there is also improvement objectively.

When the results of the portable monitoring testing are found to be satisfactory, there should also be adequate resolution of the symptoms that were present before the use of the oral appliance. When symptoms continue to be present, it may be due to other coexisting sleep disorders and not due to the sleep-disordered breathing. This is possibly the case with conditions such as sleep bruxism, insomnia, and PLM disorder. In these cases, the portable monitoring data may indicate improvement of the sleep apnea, which requires the investigation of other coexisting sleep disorders, often requiring a referral to the sleep medicine specialist.

The use of the portable monitor offers advantages that allow for ongoing assessment of the impact of the oral appliance that cannot be assessed through simple questioning of the patient. By testing at various intervals in the treatment/titration process, the oral appliance can be adjusted and modified based on both subjective as well as objective data. In addition, the issue of improving the nasal airway during sleep can be ongoing in an effort to minimize or eliminate any mouth breathing, and as that therapy progresses the portable monitor will be able to assess the impact on the sleep apnea and how well the oral appliance is performing.

Advantages to use of the level 3 portable monitor include:

1. Ease of use by both the patient and the doctor
2. Cost-effective for determination of the need for oral appliance adjustment and modification (titration)
3. Testing can be done on multiple occasions to allow for ongoing titration of the oral appliance before a more detailed sleep study
4. Results of the study are quickly available.

Disadvantages to use of the level 3 portable monitor include:

1. A lead may come loose and data are lost or not recorded
2. Device may simply not record properly
3. Device may be turned off or be taken off during sleep and thus there are no data recorded
4. Cost of disposables may be a factor in the per test cost
5. Patient may have difficulty hooking up the portable monitor.

The assessment of the successful effect of the oral appliance using portable monitoring may not be totally accurate based on the limitations of these devices as well as the specific limitations of the patient and of coexisting sleep disorders. For these reasons, the outcome of the level 3 portable monitoring study should be shared with the sleep medicine specialist and the patient's primary care physician. The clinical guidelines indicate that when level 3 portable monitors are being used for diagnosis, the results need to be interpreted by a sleep medicine specialist. However, when these same devices are being used for titration, the need for interpreting the results is not defined. At this point, the resolution of the validity of this would best be achieved by a clinical study where an oral appliance is being used that compares the simultaneous use of the level 3 portable monitor and the polysomnogram. These data would determine the usefulness of the portable monitor for titration of the oral appliance as well as its use for confirmation of the effectiveness of the oral appliance in the management of the sleep apnea.

Another issue related to the use of the portable monitor by the nonphysician, in this case the dentist, is the cost. This applies to both the cost of the device, the cost for each test, and any related billing for the testing. The initial outlay for the portable monitor may be a concern. However, this has to be considered in relation to the potential savings in time that may be derived from being able to titrate the oral appliance more effectively and hence, decrease the number of follow-up visits for adjustment and modification, and may ultimately lead to more effective treatment outcomes. The situation as it relates to the cost for each test is directly related to the ability to charge or bill for the test. It is not advisable for the dentist to bill for any type of test that involves a diagnostic code for any type of sleep study or test. However, the cost to perform each test can adequately be absorbed into the fee for either the oral appliance or for the follow-up visit, depending on the fee structure or insurance contracted rates. The cost of each test needs to be considered when evaluating the various level 3 portable monitors that are available.

SUMMARY OF THE USE OF LEVEL 3 PORTABLE MONITORING RELATED TO ORAL APPLIANCE THERAPY

The following should be considered as it applies to the use of level 3 portable monitors related to the use of oral appliances:

1. The level 3 portable monitor is not to be used for initial screening or evaluation of patients with sleep-disordered breathing, particularly and solely by the dentist, who is advocating the use of an oral appliance for the management of this condition.
2. The level 3 portable monitor can be used as an objective measurement device for the titration (adjustment and modification) of the oral appliance to achieve an optimum and effective outcome.
3. The portable monitor could be used at a future time to reevaluate the quality of sleep of the patient who is using an oral appliance when symptoms related to sleep-disordered breathing recur.
4. The portable monitor could be used to retest an oral appliance at various intervals in time to be certain that it is continuing to perform optimally. This might be done every 3 to 5 years.
5. The portable monitor can be used at the time when a replacement oral appliance is needed. It could be used to titrate the replacement oral appliance or to determine that it is functioning at the same level as the previous one. In this situation, the results of the testing would be compared with the subjective symptoms and their improvement.

6. The use of the portable monitor to evaluate the effect of the oral appliance ideally should also be able to test for sleep bruxism. A few devices currently may be able to do this but this is not part of the standard process.

These points are not meant to serve as guidelines but to begin to offer direction for the use of the level 3 portable monitor as it relates to both the dental sleep medicine practitioner and the use of oral appliances. Over time, clinical studies and continued development of level 3 portable monitors will support the development of more and better-defined guidelines and eventually will evolve into practice parameters that will better direct the use of the testing device. This will then enhance the effectiveness as well as the acceptance of oral appliances as a treatment of sleep apnea.

REFERENCES

1. Moses A. Protocol for primary treatment of snoring by dentists. Sleep Diagnosis and Therapy 2008;3(6):21–2.
2. Levendowski DJ, Morgan T, Patrickus JE, et al. In-home evaluation of efficacy and titration of a mandibular advancement device for obstructive sleep apnea. Sleep Breath 2007;11(3):139–47.
3. Collop NA, McDowell W, Boehlecke B, et al. Clinical guidelines for the use of unattended portable monitors in the diagnosis of obstructive sleep apnea in adult patients. J Clin Sleep Med 2007;3(7):737–47.
4. Bailey DR. Oral and nasal airway screening by the dentist. Sleep Med Clin 2010; 5(1):1–8.
5. Collop NA. Home sleep testing – it is not about the test. Chest 2010;138(2):245.
6. Westbrook PR, Levendowski DJ, Cvetinovic M, et al. Description and validation of the apnea risk evaluation system – a novel method to diagnose sleep apnea-hypopnea in the home. Chest 2005;128(4):2166–75.
7. Erman MK, Stewart D, Einhorn D, et al. Validation of the ApneaLink for screening of sleep apnea: a novel and simple single-channel recording device. J Clin Sleep Med 2007;3(4):387–92.
8. Chen H, Lowe AA, Bai Y, et al. Evaluation of a portable recording device (Apnea-Link) for case selection of obstructive sleep apnea. Sleep breath 2009;13:213–9.
9. Epstein LJ, Kristo D, Strollo PJ, et al. Clinical guideline for the evaluation, management and long-term care of obstructive sleep apnea in adults. J Clin Sleep Med 2009;5(3):263–76.
10. Kushida CA, Morgentahler TI, Littner MR, et al. Practice parameters for the treatment of snoring and obstructive sleep apnea with oral appliances: an update for 1995. Sleep 2006;29(2):240–3.
11. ADSM Position Paper: Dental sleep medicine & portable monitoring. Report of the ADSM board of directors in dialogue. Dialogue 2005; issue 2. p. 10–2.
12. AADSM Treatment Protocol. Updated AADSM treatment protocol: oral appliance therapy for sleep disordered breathing. Dialogue 2009; issue 3. p 10.
13. Littner MR. Ambulatory testing for adult obstructive sleep apnea for the dentist. Sleep Med Clin 2010;5(1):99–108.
14. Guimaraes KC, Drager LF, Genta PR, et al. Effects of oropharyngeal exercises on patients with moderate obstructive sleep apnea syndrome. Am J Respir Crit Care Med 2009;179:962–6.
15. McLornan P, Verrett R, Girvan T, et al. Evaluation of obstructive sleep apnea: patient's oral appliance titration protocols. Sleep Breath 2010;14:273–84 [abstract: P16].

Surgical Reconstruction of the Upper Airway for Obstructive Sleep Apnea

Ofer Jacobowitz, MD, PhD

KEYWORDS

- Obstructive sleep apnea • UPPP • Pharyngoplasty
- Tongue base • Sleep endoscopy • DISE • Airway evaluation
- Perioperative management

RATIONALE FOR SURGERY

Obstructive sleep apnea syndrome (OSA) is a common and serious medical disorder that remains difficult to treat. OSA is characterized by repetitive episodes of upper airway obstruction leading to hypoxemia and autonomic and cortical arousals. The consequences of untreated OSA are significant and include increased risk of cardiovascular disease such hypertension, atrial fibrillation, stroke, as well as diabetes, neurocognitive dysfunction, poor quality of life, motor vehicle accidents, and premature death.[1–5] Although efficacious OSA treatments such as continuous positive airway pressure (CPAP) are available, many patients do not accept chronic, nightly use of a device for sleep, and many others do not adhere to such therapy long term.[6] Surgical airway upper reconstruction is thus appropriate for certain patient populations.

The goal of surgical and medical treatment of OSA is to provide major clinical improvement and to promote survival of the patient. Because OSA is a chronic disease, cure is uncommon, and lack of cure does not imply failure.[7] CPAP is considered a clinically effective treatment of OSA even though partial adherence is common, and possibly inadequate.[8] An apnea-hypopnea index (AHI) greater than 5 was shown to be present in as many as 73% of fully CPAP-adherent patients.[9] The primary goal of surgery is to improve clinical outcome for a chronic disease and secondarily to improve the AHI, as it is a surrogate outcome measure.

Surgical treatment of OSA has been shown to result in improved survival and function in well-controlled studies. In an analysis of more than 20,000 patients with OSA in

Disclosures: None.
Hudson Valley Ear, Nose & Throat PC, 75 Crystal Run Road, Building B, Suite 220, Middletown, NY 10941, USA
E-mail address: ojacobowitz@hudsonvalleyent.com

Dent Clin N Am 56 (2012) 453–474
doi:10.1016/j.cden.2012.02.005
0011-8532/12/$ – see front matter © 2012 Elsevier Inc. All rights reserved.

Veteran's Administration, controlled for comorbidities, survival was greater with surgery than with CPAP.[10] Long-term survival was also shown to be improved with surgery in additional studies.[11,12] Cardiovascular outcome was improved in patients treated with uvulopalatopharyngoplasty (UPPP).[13] UPPP was shown to be associated with diminished motor vehicle accident risk, with a lowering of the relative risk from 9.6 to 1.3.[14] Surgery for OSA has resulted in improved quality of life, alertness, and reaction time.[15–20]

The AHI is a surrogate outcome measure for OSA, but is nonetheless used for objective treatment outcome assessment. For surgical reconstruction for the airway, data analysis is complex given the heterogeneity of procedures and mostly small series studies. Pooling of data is necessary to assess results for specific surgical techniques and for multilevel surgical interventions. In a systematic review, surgical success, as defined by reduction in the AHI of 50% or more and an AHI of less than 20, was 66%.[21] In an evidence-based medicine review of hypopharyngeal procedures for OSA, the success rate for AHI was 35% to 62% and improvement in quality of life and daytime somnolence were also noted.[22]

Which Patients Should Undergo Surgery?

Disease severity

Which patients are the best candidates for surgical intervention, those with milder or more severe OSA? Some have suggested that surgery is more suitable for mild to moderate OSA, based on AHI criteria for severity,[23] and in some cases series, patients with more severely increased AHI scores had a lower rate of surgical success, defined only by AHI reduction.[24,25] However, in other studies, preoperative AHI severity did not correlate with successful reduction of the AHI, and anatomic staging was more predictive.[26,27] Another consideration is that otherwise untreated patients with moderate to severe OSA are at higher risk for adverse sequelae, and therefore have the greatest need for treatment using surgery.

Discrete anatomic lesions

Patients with discrete anatomic loci that are amenable to surgery, such as enlarged palatine tonsils, are good candidates for surgery as the primary treatment. In the pediatric population, tonsillectomy and adenoidectomy are the recommended first-line therapies for OSA.[28] Likewise, in a young adult with palatine tonsillar hypertrophy, it is more reasonable to perform tonsillectomy than to instruct the patient to use an appliance for decades. Hypertrophic lingual tonsils, at the tongue base, are also readily amenable to simple surgical resection with resultant airway enlargement. Lingual tonsils are most commonly identified by flexible fiberoptic endoscopy performed by an otolaryngologist, and are also readily apparent on magnetic resonance imaging (MRI). Infrequently, obstructive lesions such as antrochoanal polyp, nasal or nasopharyngeal tumors, pharyngeal or laryngeal lesions, and goiters may also mediate OSA and may be surgically resected for treatment.

Nasal obstruction

Patients with nasal obstruction may find it more difficult to tolerate CPAP and oral appliance therapy. For oral appliance therapy, nasal obstruction may compromise the ability to use an appliance that partially occludes the mouth. Patients who did not respond to oral appliance therapy were shown to have higher nasal resistance compared with responders.[29] Women with complaints of nasal obstruction had an odds radio for successful treatment using oral appliances of only 0.1.[30] For CPAP use, preferential oral breathing and nasal obstruction have also been shown to be risk factors for low use and acceptance.[31,32] Nasal surgery has been shown to result in lower CPAP levels for treatment and improved adherence in small studies.[33–35] Thus nasal surgery may be used to facilitate medical therapy for OSA.

Is nasal surgery appropriate for definitive therapy for OSA? When used as the only surgical intervention, the overall success rate of septal and turbinate surgery, as defined by AHI reduction of 50% and to a level less than 20 per hour, is about 17%.[36,37] Response to nasal surgery may depend on whether there is a postoperative shift from oral breathing to more nasal breathing[37] and absence of other contributory loci for airway obstruction, often present in patients with OSA. Nasal surgery has been shown to reduce sleepiness and improve quality of life for patients with OSA, as measured by the Epworth Sleepiness Score (ESS) and Short Form 36 inventory.[38–40] These quality-of-life scores are relevant to patients with OSA and do not correlate with the AHI. Nasal surgery is thus often used in combination with pharyngeal surgery, primarily to improve quality of life.

UPPER AIRWAY EVALUATION

The upper airway is a complex space, whose dimensions and morphology are determined by skeletal and soft tissues. For anatomic analysis for surgery, it is important to conceptualize the skeletal structural container as well as the soft tissue contents. Patients with OSA have been shown to have retruded maxillae,[41] enlarged tongues, and thick pharyngeal walls,[42,43] but the presence and magnitude of anatomic features vary between patients. Hence, staging systems that describe the anatomic features are needed to target surgical intervention.

Awake, office examination is used to assess the skeletal and soft tissue features. Retrognathia, maxillary retrusion, and hard palate width are noted. The presence of oral and pharyngeal macroglossia is assessed using direct examination and fiberoptic endoscopy in the supine, end-expiratory state. The relative position of the oral tongue, presence of crenations, and central grooving are noted as markers of relative macroglossia (**Fig. 1**). The width of the oropharynx, presence of soft palatal webbing, and tonsillar size are assessed. The tongue base is examined for lingual tonsillar size the presence of lesions, glossoptosis, and epiglottic morphology (**Fig. 2**). Some surgeons use the Mueller maneuver, consisting of negative pressure against a closed mouth and nose to assess for hypopharyngeal collapse.

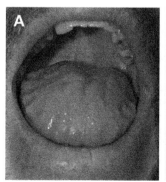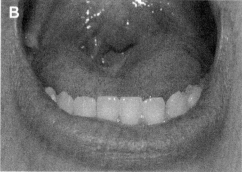

Fig. 1. Macroglossia. (*A*) The tongue is above the occlusal plane, with lateral crenations and the margin of the soft palate is not seen. (*B*) The tongue is above the occlusal plane, with lateral crenations, and has central grooving.

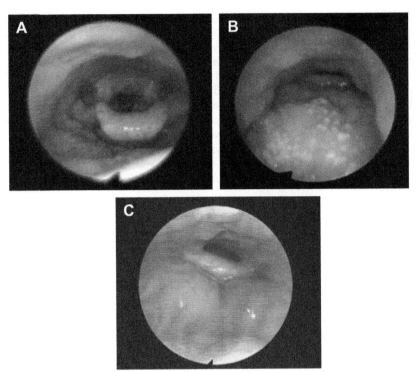

Fig. 2. Tongue base/hypopharynx: transnasal endoscopic examination. (*A*) Patent hypopharynx. The larynx is fully seen and the tongue base is minimally visible in the lower margin of the photograph. (*B*) Glossoptosis. The tongue base occupies the field of view and only the epiglottis is seen superiorly in the photograph. (*C*) Markedly large lingual tonsils are seen displacing the epiglottis.

A commonly used surgical staging system is the Friedman tongue position,[44] a modification of the Malampatti scale, in which the tongue position is assessed in reference to the soft palate (**Fig. 3**). When the tongue position is combined with tonsillar size and body mass index (BMI), the Friedman staging system may be used to predict patient success with traditional UPPP surgery. Patients with smaller tongues and larger tonsils have a high rate of success, as defined by the AHI, for UPPP with tonsillectomy. However, this system does not describe the pharyngeal morphology or airway shape and does not direct specific airway procedures; it only specifies a pharyngeal level.

A more recent anatomic system for the awake patient was proposed by Woodson,[45] incorporating the luminal shape and underlying structural features of the upper airway (**Fig. 4**). For example, the retropalatal pharyngeal airway is assessed in terms of its width, anteroposterior length, and overall shape. Taken together with knowledge of the structures that determine different pharyngeal shapes, the surgeon may then elect to perform a specific palatopharyngoplasty procedure variant. For example, if a flat/vertical airway shape is noted, consistent with anteroposterior narrowing of the superior retropalatal airway, then procedures that advance the superior palate anteriorly are selected, rather than a distal palate, soft tissue UPPP. If a circular/deep airway shape is noted, then the surgeon may select procedures that modify the distal soft palate and the thickened lateral pharyngeal wall, as described later in this article.

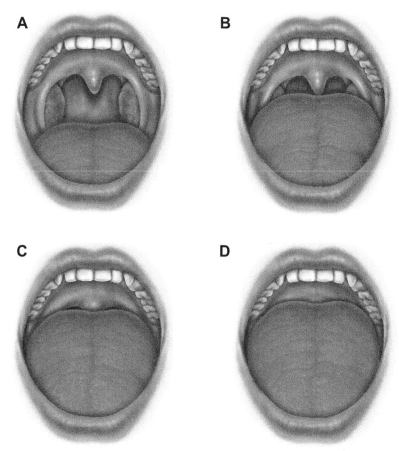

Fig. 3. Friedman tongue position. Tongue position relative to the palate is staged from A to D. (*A*) Complete visualization of uvula and tonsillar pillars; (*B*) complete visualization of uvula and partial view of tonsillar pillars and tonsils; (*C*) visualization of soft palate but not the uvula; (*D*) visualization of hard palate only. (*From* Friedman D, Ibrahim H, Bass L. Clinical staging for sleep-disordered breathing. Otolaryngol Head Neck Surg 2002;127:13–21; with permission.)

Drug-induced Sleep Endoscopy

To better approximate the airway examination during sleep, drug-induced sleep endoscopy (DISE) may be used for preoperative assessment. Infusion of agents such as propofol or midazolam is used to induce snoring and airway instability, as muscle tone is reduced with sedation. Snoring occurs in patients with OSA but not in control subjects,[46,47] and the technique has been shown to result in similar AHI levels as in true sleep except that rapid eye movement is diminished or absent in DISE and thus may not be as reliable for REM-dependent OSA. Using sedated, sleep endoscopy, operative management and procedural selection has been reported to significantly change from that planned using the awake examination.[48,49] DISE has been also used to assess residual loci of obstruction after unsuccessful initial upper airway surgery[50] and potentially predict oral appliance treatment success.[51] Recently, Hohenhorst and colleagues[52] described a classification, to uniformly describe DISE patterns of obstruction at the velum, oropharynx, tongue base, and epiglottis (VOTE).

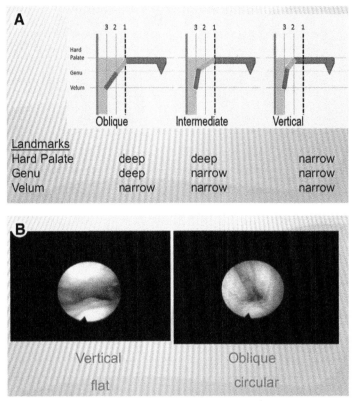

Fig. 4. (*A*) Vertical palatal sagittal view: configurations of vertical, intermediate, and obliquely oriented palates are schematically presented with corresponding anteroposterior distance at landmarks. (*B*) Corresponding endoscopic view and vertical and oblique palatal shapes. Note proximal anterior-posterior narrowing at arrowhead with flat shape and relative anterior-posterior patency with oblique shape. (*From* Woodson BT, Sitton M, Jacobowitz O. Expansion sphincter pharyngoplasty and palatal advancement pharyngoplasty: airway evaluation and surgical techniques. Oper Tech Otolaryngol 2012;23:3–10; with permission.)

PERIOPERATIVE MANAGEMENT

Patients with OSA may be at higher risk when undergoing surgery, especially on the upper airway. Before surgery, patients should undergo a thorough medical optimization given the increased risk of cardiovascular disease with OSA. Communication or consultation with the anesthesiologist is recommended because patients with OSA are often more difficult to intubate and may have a lower threshold to opiates or sedatives for respiratory depression and airway collapse. After surgery, nonsupine positioning and head elevation are preferable. Pain should be adequately controlled but use of opiates should be minimized. A multimodal regimen consisting of systemic steroids, gabapentinoids, acetaminophen, cyclooxygenase-2 selective inhibitors, antibiotics, and tissue cooling may be used to treat and prevent pain, to lower the opiate requirement for analgesia.[53] Patients are typically observed several hours or in an inpatient setting, depending on specific procedures performed, medical comorbidities, and OSA severity.

SURGICAL PROCEDURE SELECTION

Although UPPP is the most common procedure performed for OSA, the range of upper and lower pharyngeal procedures that are used to address the upper airway is extensive. A nonexhaustive list in presented in **Table 1**, in which procedures are grouped based on sites. The choice of procedure depends on patient features, the surgeon's expertise, and patient preferences. There is no widely accepted protocol in the sleep surgery community for airway reconstruction. The Stanford protocol of Riley and Powell[24] has been of great value but is limited because it only includes UPPP, genioglossus advancement, hyoid suspension as phase I, maxillomandibular advancement as phase II, and because this multiprocedure protocol is of high intensity and morbidity.

Patients may undergo staged or concurrent procedures for upper airway reconstruction depending on their personal preferences or those of their surgeon. From a safety perspective, performance of nasal with upper pharyngeal surgery does not seem to increase the risk for serious complications but concurrent upper pharyngeal and hypopharyngeal surgeries are of higher risk.[54] From the patient's perspective, concurrent surgery may be preferred given the convenience of only 1 operative event and work hiatus. However, others may prefer staged surgeries that may be performed ambulatory, with less pain, and more rapid return to work. Another reason why staged surgery may be preferable is that the preoperative assessment of procedures needed for effective therapy is not always accurate and that a single procedure, rather than multiple procedures, may suffice.

Table 1
Upper airway surgical procedures for OSA

Site	Procedure
Nasal/nasopharyngeal	Septoplasty Inferior turbinate reduction Nasal valve repair Nasal valve suspension Nasal polypectomy Adenoidectomy
Oral	Tongue ablation Lingualplasty Excision of oral tori
Oropharyngeal	Uvulopalatopharyngoplasty Lateral pharyngoplasty Palatal advancement pharyngoplasty Z-palatopharyngoplasty Relocation pharyngoplasty Anterior pharyngoplasty Tonsillectomy
Hypopharyngeal	Partial glossectomy Radiofrequency tongue ablation Lingual tonsillectomy Genioglossus advancement Tongue suspension Epiglottoplasty
Neck	Hyoid suspension Tracheotomy
Multilevel	Maxillomandibular advancement

The difficulty in predicting a priori the extent of surgery needed may be related to postoperative changes in pharyngeal pressures, anatomic palate-tongue interaction, or neuromuscular tone differences not apparent during an examination while awake. Surgery on the upper pharynx may affect the lower pharynx and vice versa. In patients who underwent palatal surgery, the degree of subpalatal obstructions was lower after surgery, as measured by manometry.[55] The potential mechanism may be that, after alleviation of the upper pharyngeal critical obstruction, lower overall negative pharyngeal pressures are generated and less tongue base obstruction occurs. An additional palatal-tongue relation is anatomic. Recent study showed anatomic connection of the superior constrictor muscle with the tongue's transversus intrinsic muscle,[56] hence tongue or palatal modification may affect the latter as well.

The author's current preference is to perform staged surgeries rather than more intensive multilevel concurrent procedures. Although a prior protocol consisting of UPPP, genioglossus advancement, hyoid suspension, and radiofrequency treatment of the tongue base resulted in symptomatic treatment and AHI reduction to less than 20 with greater than 50% reduction from baseline for 74% of patients of an advanced Friedman stage, the approach was associated with high morbidity.[57] Procedures are now performed staged, and patients with moderate to severe OSA are observed overnight for airway and cardiovascular monitoring, and treated using a multimodal analgesia protocol. A palatopharyngoplasty procedure is usually performed first, because the upper pharyngeal airway is the narrowest site in the upper airway and, with treatment, downstream hypopharyngeal collapse could diminish. About 3 months following surgery, patients are assessed using sleep studies for the need for subsequent intervention before proceeding with additional surgery.

PROCEDURES
Nasal

Inferior turbinate reduction
The inferior turbinate may contribute to anterior nasal obstruction, especially in the setting of allergic or nonallergic chronic rhinitis. If medical therapy such as topical nasal steroid spray use does not result in sufficient airway improvement, surgical treatment may be performed consisting of turbinate reduction and/or lateralization (outfracturing). In the past, the anterior portion of the turbinate was simply trimmed but this approach was associated with pain, bleeding, prolonged crusting, and potential for nasal dryness (ozena). Modern methods include submucosal turbinate reduction performed through a tiny incision at the head of turbinate using microdebriders, radiofrequency probes, bipolar cautery, or manual cutting forceps. Using current methods, risks are minimal and procedures may be performed under local anesthesia or sedation in the office or operating room and postoperative nasal packing is rarely used. The microdebrider technique may be preferable because it allows removal of conchal bone as well as soft tissue.

Septoplasty
A deviated septum may severely narrow the nasal airway (**Fig. 5**). Septoplasty techniques can vary greatly between patients, depending on the location of the deviation and the need for release of septal attachments. The septal cartilage and bone are accessed through an anterior incision and, most commonly, spurs and misshaped segments are excised. When the anterior-caudal septum is mediating the obstruction, incisional techniques and sometimes grafting are used because this portion of the septum is vital for tip stability. When the inferior or superior septal attachments are contributing to the obstruction, releasing cuts are performed with subsequent suture

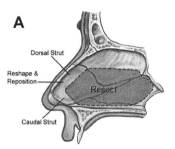
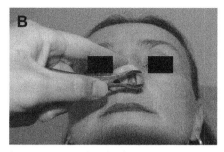

Fig. 5. The nasal septum. (*A*) To repair an obstructive septal deformity, excision may be performed in the region marked as resect but, caudally and dorsally, repositioning and contouring is performed to preserve form and stability. (*B*) Severe caudal septal deviation. ([*A*] *From* Golde A. Rhinoplastic techniques for the nasal valve for the patient with sleep apnea. Oper Tech Otolaryngol 2006;17:242–251; with permission.)

stabilization of the septum in the midline. Septoplasty is performed under general anesthesia or sedation and usually does not require nasal packing.

Nasal valve surgery

Nasal valve surgery includes a variety of techniques to address narrowing and/or collapse of the internal or external nasal valves. The external nasal valve is the nostril or alar airway. This area may be narrowed medially by septal deflection, the medial crura of the alar cartilages, and superior-laterally by loss of structural support of the alar lobule (**Fig. 6**). Cartilage grafting techniques may be used to provide structural support to the weakened structures. Excisional, incisional, and repositioning procedures are used to modify the shape of the alar airway and address the obstructive elements.

The internal nasal valve is at the junction of the head of the inferior turbinate with the caudal portion of the upper lateral cartilage superior-laterally and the septum medially. If treatment of the septum is inadequate to expand the valve, cartilage grafting is often used to widen the valve (spreader grafts) or to tent up weak lateral nasal wall and thereby enlarge the valve region. An intranasal Z-plasty technique is also used by some to widen the valve.

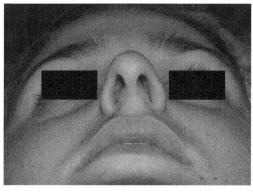

Fig. 6. External nasal valve stenosis. Splayed medial crura of the alar cartilage and weak lateral alae contribute to obstruction.

The pyriform aperture may be narrow in patients with OSA because they commonly have an underdeveloped maxilla. Lateral expansion may be simply performed using a small intranasal incision and bone removal using a microdebrider, bur, or rongeur.

The nasal valve may also collapse with inspiration. To stabilize the valve, rhinoplasty overlay grafting may be used, but simpler suture suspension may also be performed. Minimally invasive suspension techniques involve suture passage around the supero-lateral collapse zone with suspension to a bone-anchor microscrew inserted into the maxilla infraorbitally through a tiny incision or simply by passing the suture through small drill holes in the piriform rim intransally (**Fig. 7**).

Oropharyngeal Procedures

Palatopharyngoplasty techniques consist of surgical modification of the soft palate and pharyngeal walls with or without tonsillectomy. UPPP is a common term used to refer to such procedures, in which some distal soft palate tissue resection is performed and suture suspension is used to suspend the palate and expand the pharyngeal airway (**Fig. 8**). However, UPPP is a poor term because the procedure can vary between surgeons, and even when performed in different patients by the same surgeon.

In recent years, procedures have been developed to address specific airway morphologies and structures more precisely. These procedures include the expansion sphincter pharyngoplasty of Pang and Woodson[58] and the lateral pharyngoplasty of Cahali and colleagues,[59] the transpalatal advancement pharyngoplasty of Woodson,[45,60] the Z-palatoplasty of Friedman,[61] and the relocation pharyngoplasty of Li.[62] Laser-assisted uvulopalatopharyngoplasty (LAUP) is no longer frequently used because of questionable effectiveness, associated pain, and the potential for pharyngeal stenosis. Another recent trend by some surgeons is to preserve the uvula because it serves to lubricate and channel flow into the pharynx and its resection is

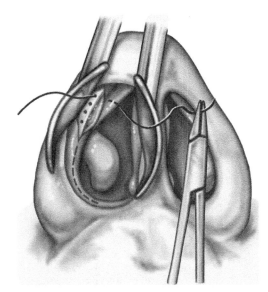

Fig. 7. Nasal valve stabilization technique. A suspension suture is passed around the upper lateral cartilage and through drill holes in the piriform rim. The suture is tied to stabilize the internal nasal valve. (*From* Weaver EM. Nasal valve stabilization. Oper Tech Otolaryngol 2012;23:59–63; with permission.)

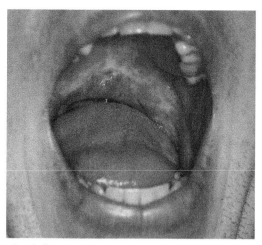

Fig. 8. UPPP/uvulopalatal flap. A UPPP procedure was performed. The uvula was not resected, but rotated and sutured anterosuperiorly.

associated with symptoms such as globus, pharyngeal dryness, and thickened secretions.

Expansion sphincter pharyngoplasty (lateral pharyngoplasty)

The lateral pharyngeal wall is thickened or medialized in many patients with OSA. Lateral pharyngoplasty techniques were developed to address this pattern of obstruction, as described by Cahali and colleagues,[59] Li,[62] and Pang and Woodson.[58] The expansion sphincter pharyngoplasty technique was described by Pang and Woodson.[58] The palatopharyngeus muscle is identified in the tonsillar fossa and released only inferiorly. The muscle is then rotated superiorly, anteriorly, and laterally through a submucosal tunnel and secured by suture to the hamular periosteum (**Fig. 9**). This procedure results in debulking of the lateral wall as well as lateral and anterior pharyngeal expansion mediated by the posterior and superior attachment of the palatopharyngeus to the superior constrictor muscle and to the palate. Additional procedures on the soft palate, tonsils, and uvula may be added as needed.

Transpalatal advancement pharyngoplasty Transpalatal advancement pharyngoplasty (TAP),[45] developed by B.T. Woodson, is used to expand the pharyngeal airway narrowed in the anterior-posterior direction. It is particularly suitable for patients with superior retropalatal obstruction and can expand this region. UPPP-type resection of distal palatal soft tissue cannot achieve expansion of a narrow superior pharyngeal isthmus. TAP may also be combined with additional procedures on the soft palate, tonsils, and uvula as needed. It is also useful to perform after conventional UPPP failure. After exposure of the hard palate and removal of torus palatini, a segment of 8 to 10 mm of bone from the posterior hard palate is burred away, leaving about a 2-mm segment of palatine bone attached to the soft palate. The soft palate and attached bony strip are mobilized anteriorly following lateral osteotomies and tensor veli palatini aponeurotic cuts. The advancement is secured using multiple sutures passed through anterior drill holes in the hard palate, circumscribing the bony strip or resuspending the tensor aponeurosis (**Fig. 10**). The procedure is effective at expanding the pharyngeal airway, causes only mild-moderate pain, but carries the risk of fistula.

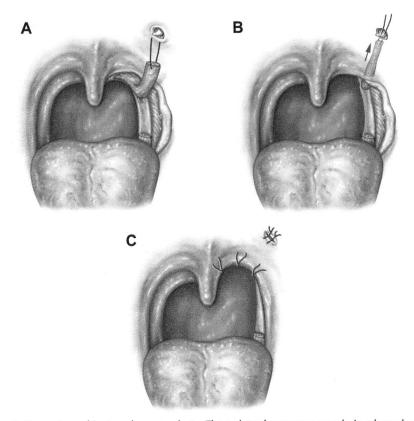

Fig. 9. Expansion sphincter pharyngoplasty. The palatopharyngeus muscle is released only inferiorly (*A*) and is then rotated superiorly, anteriorly, and laterally through a submucosal tunnel (*B*) and secured by suture to the hamular periosteum (*C*). (*From* Woodson BT, Sitton M, Jacobowitz O. Expansion sphincter pharyngoplasty and palatal advancement pharyngoplasty: airway evaluation and surgical techniques. Oper Tech Otolaryngol 2012;23:3–10; with permission.)

Z-palatoplasty Z-palatoplasty is an aggressive palatopharyngoplasty developed by Friedman and colleagues[61] that may also be used to treat failure at the retropalatal region following conventional UPPP. The soft palate and uvula are transected in the midline to the mid–soft palate vertically. The palatoglossus and palatopharyngeus muscles are also transected superiorly. The 2 palatal flaps are then rotated from the midline anteriorly, laterally, and superiorly and sutured in place (**Fig. 11**). The procedure results in anterior and lateral pharyngeal expansion and a favorable direction for scar contracture. However, it is associated with higher rates of velopharyngeal insufficiency.

Hypopharyngeal Procedures

Hypopharyngeal obstruction may occur because of tongue bulk, lingual tonsils, glossoptosis, epiglottic/supraglottic collapse, or lateral pharyngeal wall medialization. Cold-steel or electrocautery techniques for the tongue base were associated with potential for airway edema and pain and have mostly been replaced with techniques using radiofrequency ablation or suspension.

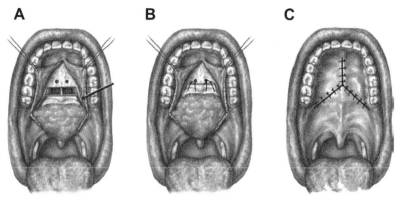

Fig. 10. Transpalatal advancement pharyngoplasty. (*A*) The hard palate is exposed with the resected segment and anterior palatal drill holes shown. (*B*) Suspension sutures are passed through the drill holes and around the posterior osteotomy segment medially as well as through the tensor tendon aponeurosis laterally. (*C*) The mucosal incision is approximated. (*From* Woodson BT, Sitton M, Jacobowitz O. Expansion sphincter pharyngoplasty and palatal advancement pharyngoplasty: airway evaluation and surgical techniques. Oper Tech Otolaryngol 2012;23:3–10; with permission.)

Radiofrequency tongue ablation/partial glossectomy

Temperature-controlled radiofrequency ablation (TCRF) of the tongue base was developed to reduce the pain and edema associated with conventional resection. Radiofrequency probes are inserted into the tongue and tongue base after local

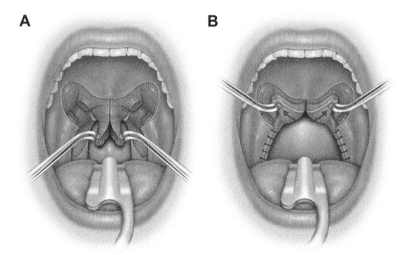

Fig. 11. Z-palatoplasty. (*A*) Anterior exposure of the soft palate is shown after mucosal removal. The uvula and soft palate are divided in the midline to the mid–soft palate vertically. (*B*) Following division of the palatoglossus and palatopharyngeus muscles, the 2 palatal flaps are rotated anteriorly, laterally, and superiorly and sutured in place. (*Modified from* Friedman M, Wilson M, Kelley K. Z-palatoplasty technique and review of five-year experience. Oper Tech Otolaryngol 2012;23:22–7; with permission.)

anesthetic injection and thermal lesions are produced at multiple locations. This technique was performed under local anesthesia, and resulted in significant functional improvement for patients with OSA, mild reduction in the AHI in a placebo-controlled study,[15] and small tongue base reduction.

An excisional technique using the Coblation device has largely replaced the TCRF technique because Coblation allows large volumetric tongue reduction with low morbidity compared with older glossectomy techniques.[63] The procedure is performed transorally, using angled rigid telescopes for visualization and a malleable radiofrequency bipolar handpiece (**Fig. 12**). Tissue cooling is achieved using saline irrigation and thereby ablation occurs at low temperature. Traction sutures are used to advance the tongue and provide improved exposure. Both submucosal (tunnel) and transmucosal techniques have been used. Ultrasound localization of the neurovascular bundle may be performed to guide the surgeon to the limits of resection, and some identify the bundle to perform more aggressive resection. The Coblation device may also be used to perform oral tongue reduction, although care must be taken to avoid neurovascular injury.

Recently, transoral robot-assisted surgical (TORS) resection of the tongue base has been performed. The da Vinci (Intuitive Surgical, Sunnyvale, CA) robotic system allows improved visualization, magnification, and multiple degrees of freedom for tissue manipulation. This approach is currently being studied and seems promising. Although theoretically advantageous, it is not known whether TORS is preferable to endoscopic tongue base ablation with respect to effectiveness and morbidity.

Lingual tonsillectomy

Lingual tonsillectomy can be performed using Coblation for hypertrophic lingual tonsils.[63] Resection may be performed endoscopically with low morbidity. For exposure, often a midline tongue furrow is first created. Recently, TORS has been used for excision of lingual tonsils.

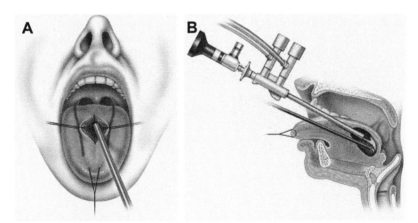

Fig. 12. Midline glossectomy. (*A*) Transoral midline glossectomy is performed using the Coblation device. The tongue is pulled anteriorly using sutures for improved exposure while tissue dissolution is performed medial to the neurovascular bundles. (*B*) Sagittal view of submucosal midline glossectomy, performed with rigid endoscope visualization. Alternatively, the procedure may be performed through a more posterior midline trench. (*From* Robinson S. Chapter 47: External submucosal glossectomy. In: Friedman M, editor. Sleep apnea and snoring: surgical and non-surgical therapy. Philadelphia: Saunders/Elsevier; 2009. p. 292–300; with permission.)

Genioglossus advancement

Genioglossus advancement has been extensively used in multilevel protocols for OSA since its introduction by Riley and colleagues[64] in the 1980s.[24] A mucosal incision is performed in the lower lip from premolar to premolar and exposure of the labial surface of the mandible is obtained. The location of the genial tubercle is estimated by palpation and radiograph review (panoramic and periapical). A rectangular horizontal osteotomy is performed below the dental apices, spanning the width of the lower incisors and about 1 cm in height. The osteotomy segment, attached to the genioglossus muscles, is mobilized forward and the bone is thinned until only the lingual cortex remains. The osteotomy segment is then rotated less than 90° to achieve overlap of the mandible surface to permit fixation with a single screw (**Fig. 13**). Incisions are then closed, ice is applied, and the patient is observed on the ward for edema of the floor of the mouth . Dental paresthesias and, rarely, vascular compromise of the incisors may occur.

Tongue suspension

Tongue suspension has been used for patients with OSA with glossoptosis most often in combination with palatopharyngoplasty, with improved outcome compared with pharyngoplasty alone. Because a suture is used for suspension, degradation or breakage of the suture may occur and efficacy may decrease in the long term.[65] The technique may be performed using a floor of mouth incision or small submental incision. A 5-mm titanium screw is inserted into the lingual cortex of the mandible using the AIRvance, formerly known as the Repose tool (Medtronic, Minneapolis, MN). Polypropylene sutures, attached to the screw, are passed using a trocar in a superior to posterior direction through the submental incision onto the tongue dorsum. The sutures are submucosalized and the triangular suture tract is tightened as the suture is tied. Tongue edema and pain are potential risks.

Epiglottoplasty

The epiglottis may collapse medially or posteriorly, as seen during DISE. Partial epiglottic resection, stiffening, and adhesion may be performed using laser, Coblation, and TORS. In the author's experience, epiglottic procedures are performed in later-stage surgery, because relief of upstream obstruction may reduce the pressure gradient for downstream epiglottic collapse and obviate need for epiglottic surgery.

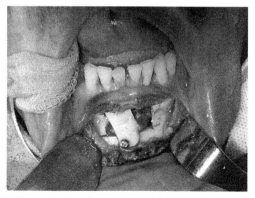

Fig. 13. Genioglossus advancement. The osteotomy fragment is shown rotated and fixed to the labial surface of the mandible. The genioglossus muscle is shown within the bone window, drawn anteriorly.

Cervical Procedures

Hyoid suspension

The hyoid suspension was introduced by Riley and colleagues[24] as part of their phase 1 multilevel surgery protocol for OSA. The initial technique was a hyomandibular suspension but hyolaryngeal suspension is also performed. The rationale for advancing the hyoid is that it serves as an attachment point to muscles including the hyoglossus, genioglossus, geniohyoid, and middle constrictor. The mechanism by which hyoid suspension aids in the treatment of OSA is uncertain and may be related to change in muscle tone or tension, epiglottic advancement, or shortening of airway length. The optimal direction of suspension is unknown and it has been proposed that hyomandibular suspension is preferred in women.[66] The procedure may be performed under sedation or general anesthesia, but sedation is advantageous because inferior and superior hyoid traction may be tried to assess airway effect before suspension (B. Woodson, personal communication and author's experience, 2006). A heavy needle or blunt suture passer (the author's preference) is used to circumscribe the hyoid in paramedian positions bilaterally and suspension is performed by suture passage through the thyroid cartilage or by suspension to the mandible via a screw (AIRvance/Repose) or drill hole . After surgery, patients may have temporary swallow dysfunction.

Tracheotomy

Tracheotomy is an upper airway bypass procedure that is highly effective but rarely accepted by patients. Before the introduction of CPAP therapy, tracheotomy was the treatment method for OSA. For patients who accept the procedure, a formal tracheostomy procedure is performed, with creation of a large stoma using skin-lined flaps. The stoma or tracheostomy tube, if used, may be occluded in the daytime for normal phonation and olfaction.

Multilevel Maxilomandibular Advancement

Maxilomandibular advancement (MMA) is a bilateral, sagittal, mandibular split osteotomy performed concurrently with a Le Fort I maxillary osteotomy, followed by advancement and fixation (**Fig. 14**). By definition, it is a multilevel surgical approach, used to treat moderate to severe OSA by jaw advancement. MMA is phase 2 of the Stanford protocol for OSA but may also be performed outright without prior procedures. Effectiveness of MMA is high, supported by multiple concordant case series.[67] Malocclusion is not often corrected before surgery given the urgency to treat and the suboptimal status of dentition and gingiva in many patients with OSA, as well as the cost. The procedure is usually performed in younger adult patients, and may not be as effective in obese patients. The procedure is intensive and not frequently accepted by patients. Hypoesthesia of the chin and lip often occurs and may be permanent in 9% to 85% of cases.[68] Patients frequently also undergo prolonged oral rehabilitation for trismus and occlusion.

Future Directions

Hypoglossal neurostimulation (HGN) is an experimental method for OSA treatment[69,70] that is currently in US Food and Drug Administration trials. The rationale for the treatment is that increased tongue muscle tone and pharyngeal stiffness maintain a narrowed airway patent during wakefulness and during sleep, whereas loss of muscle tone leads to pharyngeal obstruction. Following implantation of a pulse generator capable of stimulating the hypoglossal nerve, the patient is treated by activating the stimulator using a remote controller before sleep. This option may appeal for

A   B

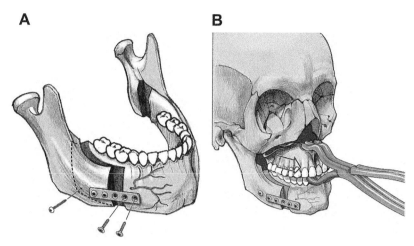

Fig. 14. Maxillomandibular advancement. (*A*) Following mandibular split osteotomy, the anterior segment is advanced at least 10 mm and plated. (*B*) The maxilla is advanced anteriorly following Le Fort I osteotomy. (*From* Blumen M, Vezina JP, Pigot JL, et al. Maxillomandibular advancement for obstructive sleep apnea syndrome. Oper Tech Otolaryngol 2012;23:63; with permission.)

patients who do not tolerate a CPAP interface or intraoral appliance. Three different devices are currently being tested. Inspire (Minneapolis, MN, USA) and Apnex's (St Paul, MN, USA) HGN schemes include implantation of a respiratory sensing lead in addition to the pulse generator and hypoglossal nerve electrode in order to couple phasic stimulation to the breathing phase. Imthera's scheme (San Diego, CA, USA) obviates a respiratory sensing lead, instead using tonic stimulation cycled among multiple contacts of the electrode to prevent muscle fatigue.

CASES

1. A 59-year-old teacher presented with poor sleep, chronic loud snoring, and chronic fatigue. On physical examination, he had a BMI of 30, severe hard palate narrowing, overbite, tongue position of about 3, severe lateral pharyngeal narrowing, and septal deviation. By polysomnography, he had an AHI of 83, lowest oxygen saturation (LSAT) of 76%, and multiple premature ventricular contractions (PVCs). He had tried CPAP at 7 to 8 cm of pressure but reported discomfort and was unable to sleep well. Oral appliance therapy was tried but he snored even at 6 cm advancement from 60% protrusive position. On DISE, he had marked medial pharyngeal wall collapse. Expansion sphincter pharyngoplasty was performed (**Fig. 15**) with overnight observation. He had mild pain after surgery. Three months after surgery, he reported improved daytime function and sleep quality, and snoring was mild. On polysomnogram, he had an AHI of 3 and LSAT of 88%, and no PVCs were noted.
2. A 50-year-old teacher presented with poor sleep, chronic loud snoring, nasal obstruction, and excessive daytime sleepiness. On physical examination he had a BMI of 34, malocclusion class 3, tongue position of 4, severe lateral pharyngeal narrowing, and severe septal deviation. By polysomnography (split-night study), he had an AHI of 51, left AHI of 57, and LSAT of 83%. He had unsuccessfully tried treatment using CPAP at 15 cm of pressure and a thermoplastic oral appliance. A staged surgical plan consisting of nasal, tongue, and lateral pharyngeal surgery

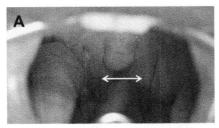
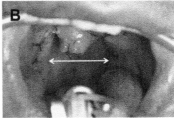

Fig. 15. Expansion sphincter pharyngoplasty. (*A*) The patient's preoperative oropharynx is shown, with the tongue depressed using a surgical retractor. The pharyngeal width, indicated by white arrows, is highly narrowed. Pharyngeal depth is also minimal. (*B*) At the completion of the procedure, pharyngeal width, indicated by white arrows, is markedly greater. Pharyngeal depth is greater, as noted by the anterior soft palate position.

was proposed for his multiple obstructive elements. On DISE, he had marked medial pharyngeal wall collapse, concentric velopharyngeal collapse, and macroglossia. Coblation partial (midline) glossectomy, septoplasty, and turbinate reduction were performed with overnight observation. He had mild to moderate pain after surgery. He then used CPAP at a lower level of 10 cm H_2O but opted for lateral pharyngoplasty given partial symptomatic improvement after the initial surgery. Immediately before undergoing expansion sphincter pharyngoplasty, DISE was performed in which the hypopharynx appeared patent but marked medial pharyngeal wall and concentric velopharyngeal collapse were present. Three months after surgery, he reported improved daytime alertness and sleep quality, with minimal snoring present. On a polysomnogram, he had an AHI of 8, left AHI of 6, supine AHI of 14, and LSAT of 83% (for 0.2 minutes at <90% saturation).

SUMMARY

Surgical therapy for OSA is a complex but potentially effective treatment of the patient with OSA. Patients with mild to severe OSA who fail noninvasive treatment, or patients with discrete anatomic lesions, are good candidates for surgery. Upper airway assessment for surgery is performed in the office while the patient is awake as well as using DISE to identify the loci and structural targets for surgical reconstruction. Careful perioperative management is needed to minimize airway and cardiovascular risk. Surgical procedures may be performed staged or concurrently, but staging may be better tolerated. Surgical techniques have evolved to more precisely target specific anatomic structures and patterns of pharyngeal collapse, rather than to treat levels of obstruction. Future directions in surgical therapy include the use of robotic tools and hypoglossal neurostimulation.

REFERENCES

1. Yaggi HK, Concato J, Kernan WN, et al. Obstructive sleep apnea as a risk factor for stroke and death. N Engl J Med 2005;353:2034–41.
2. Marin JM, Carrizo SJ, Vicente E, et al. Long-term cardiovascular outcomes in men with obstructive sleep apnoea-hypopnoea with or without treatment with continuous positive airway pressure: an observational study. Lancet 2005;365:1046–53.
3. Gami AS, Pressman G, Caples SM, et al. Association of atrial fibrillation and obstructive sleep apnea. Circulation 2004;110:364–7.

4. Naegele B, Thouvard V, Pepin JL, et al. Deficits of cognitive executive functions in patients with sleep apnea syndrome. Sleep 1995;18:43–52.

5. Ellen RL, Marshall SC, Palayew M. Systematic review of motor vehicle crash risk in persons with sleep apnea. J Clin Sleep Med 2006;2:193–200.

6. Richard W, Venker J, den Herder C, et al. Acceptance and long-term compliance of nCPAP in obstructive sleep apnea. Eur Arch Otorhinolaryngol 2007;264:1081–6.

7. Weaver EM. Judging sleep apnea surgery. Sleep Med Rev 2010;14:283–5.

8. Ravesloot MJ, de Vries N. Reliable calculation of the efficacy of non-surgical and surgical treatment of obstructive sleep apnea revisited. Sleep 2011;34:105–10.

9. Pittman SD, Pillar G, Berry RB, et al. Follow-up assessment of CPAP efficacy in patients with obstructive sleep apnea using an ambulatory device based on peripheral arterial tonometry. Sleep Breath 2006;10:123–31.

10. Weaver EM, Maynard C, Yueh B. Survival of veterans with sleep apnea: continuous positive airway pressure versus surgery. Otolaryngol Head Neck Surg 2004;130(6):659–65.

11. Keenan SP, Burt H, Ryan CF, et al. Long-term survival of patients with obstructive sleep apnea treated by uvulopalatopharyngoplasty or nasal CPAP. Chest 1994;105:155–9.

12. Marti S, Sampol G, Munoz X, et al. Mortality in severe sleep apnoea/hypopnoea syndrome patients: impact of treatment. Eur Respir J 2002;20:1511–8.

13. Peker Y, Carlson J, Hedner J. Increased incidence of coronary artery disease in sleep apnoea: a long-term follow-up. Eur Respir J 2006;28:596–602.

14. Haraldsson PO, Carenfelt C, Lysdahl M, et al. Does uvulopalatopharyngoplasty inhibit automobile accidents? Laryngoscope 1995;105:657–61.

15. Woodson BT, Steward DL, Weaver EM, et al. A randomized trial of temperature-controlled radiofrequency, continuous positive airway pressure, and placebo for obstructive sleep apnea syndrome. Otolaryngol Head Neck Surg 2003;128:848–61.

16. Steward DL, Weaver EM, Woodson BT. Multilevel temperature-controlled radiofrequency for obstructive sleep apnea: extended follow-up. Otolaryngol Head Neck Surg 2005;132:630–5.

17. Weaver EM, Woodson BT, Yueh B, et al. Studying Life Effects & Effectiveness of Palatopharyngoplasty (SLEEP) study: subjective outcomes of isolated uvulopalatopharyngoplasty. Otolaryngol Head Neck Surg 2011;144:623–31.

18. Li HY, Chen NH, Shu YH, et al. Changes in quality of life and respiratory disturbance after extended uvulopalatal flap surgery in patients with obstructive sleep apnea. Arch Otolaryngol Head Neck Surg 2004;130:195–200.

19. Walker-Engström ML, Wilhelmsson B, Tegelberg A, et al. Quality of life assessment of treatment with dental appliance or UPPP in patients with mild to moderate obstructive sleep apnoea. A prospective randomized 1-year follow-up study. J Sleep Res 2000;9:303–8.

20. Robinson S, Chia M, Carney AS, et al. Upper airway reconstructive surgery long-term quality-of-life outcomes compared with CPAP for adult obstructive sleep apnea. Otolaryngol Head Neck Surg 2009;141:257–63.

21. Lin HC, Friedman M, Chang HW, et al. The efficacy of multilevel surgery of the upper airway in adults with obstructive sleep apnea/hypopnea syndrome. Laryngoscope 2008;118:902–8.

22. Kezirian EJ, Goldberg AN. Hypopharyngeal surgery in obstructive sleep apnea: an evidence-based medicine review. Arch Otolaryngol Head Neck Surg 2006;132:206–13.

23. Millman RP, Carlisle CC, Rosenberg C, et al. Simple predictors of uvulopalato-pharyngoplasty outcome in the treatment of obstructive sleep apnea. Chest 2000;118:1025–30.
24. Riley RW, Powell NB, Guilleminault C. Obstructive sleep apnea syndrome: a review of 306 consecutively treated surgical patients. Otolaryngol Head Neck Surg 1993;108:117–25.
25. Xiong YP, Yi HL, Yin SK, et al. Predictors of surgical outcomes of uvulopalatophar-yngoplasty for obstructive sleep apnea hypopnea syndrome. Otolaryngol Head Neck Surg 2011;145:1049–54.
26. Li HY, Wang PC, Lee LA, et al. Prediction of uvulopalatopharyngoplasty outcome: anatomy-based staging system versus severity-based staging system. Sleep 2006;29:1537–41.
27. Friedman M, Vidyasagar R, Bliznikas D, et al. Does severity of obstructive sleep apnea/hypopnea syndrome predict uvulopalatopharyngoplasty outcome? Laryn-goscope 2005;115:2109–13.
28. Brietzke SE, Gallagher D. The effectiveness of tonsillectomy and adenoidectomy in the treatment of pediatric obstructive sleep apnea/hypopnea syndrome: a meta-analysis. Otolaryngol Head Neck Surg 2006;134:979–84.
29. Zeng B, Ng AT, Qian J, et al. Influence of nasal resistance on oral appliance treat-ment outcome in obstructive sleep apnea. Sleep 2008;31:543–7.
30. Marklund M, Stenlund H, Franklin KA. Mandibular advancement devices in 630 men and women with obstructive sleep apnea and snoring: tolerability and predictors of treatment success. Chest 2004;125:1270–8.
31. Sugiura T, Noda A, Nakata S, et al. Influence of nasal resistance on initial accep-tance of continuous positive airway pressure in treatment for obstructive sleep apnea syndrome. Respiration 2007;74:56–60.
32. Bachour A, Maasilta P. Mouth breathing compromises adherence to nasal contin-uous positive airway pressure therapy. Chest 2004;126:1248–54.
33. Nakata S, Noda A, Yagi H, et al. Nasal resistance for determinant factor of nasal surgery in CPAP failure patients with obstructive sleep apnea syndrome. Rhinol-ogy 2005;43:296–9.
34. Friedman M, Tanyeri H, Lim JW, et al. Effect of improved nasal breathing on obstructive sleep apnea. Otolaryngol Head Neck Surg 2000;122:71–4.
35. Zonato AI, Bittencourt LR, Martinho FL, et al. Upper airway surgery: the effect on nasal continuous positive airway pressure titration on obstructive sleep apnea patients. Eur Arch Otorhinolaryngol 2006;263:481–6.
36. Verse T, Pirsig W. Impact of impaired nasal breathing on sleep-disordered breathing. Sleep Breath 2003;7:63–76.
37. Koutsourelakis I, Georgoulopoulos G, Perraki E, et al. Randomised trial of nasal surgery for fixed nasal obstruction in obstructive sleep apnoea. Eur Respir J 2008;31:110–7.
38. Verse T, Maurer JT, Pirsig W. Effect of nasal surgery on sleep-related breathing disorders. Laryngoscope 2002;112:64–8.
39. Li HY, Lin Y, Chen NH, et al. Improvement in quality of life after nasal surgery alone for patients with obstructive sleep apnea and nasal obstruction. Arch Oto-laryngol Head Neck Surg 2008;134:429–33.
40. Nakata S, Noda A, Yasuma F, et al. Effects of nasal surgery on sleep quality in obstruc-tive sleep apnea syndrome with nasal obstruction. Am J Rhinol 2008;22:59–63.
41. Dempsey JA, Skatrud JB, Jacques AJ, et al. Anatomic determinants of sleep-disordered breathing across the spectrum of clinical and nonclinical male subjects. Chest 2002;122:840–51.

42. Schwab RJ, Pasirstein M, Pierson R, et al. Identification of upper airway anatomic risk factors for obstructive sleep apnea with volumetric magnetic resonance imaging. Am J Respir Crit Care Med 2003;168:522–30.
43. Tsuiki S, Isono S, Ishikawa T, et al. Anatomical balance of the upper airway and obstructive sleep apnea. Anesthesiology 2008;108:1009–15.
44. Friedman M, Ibrahim H, Bass L. Clinical staging for sleep-disordered breathing. Otolaryngol Head Neck Surg 2002;127:13–21.
45. Woodson BT, Sitton M, Jacobowitz O. Expansion sphincter pharyngoplasty and palatal advancement pharyngoplasty: airway evaluation and surgical techniques. Oper Tech Otolaryngol Head Neck Surg 2012;23:3–10.
46. Berry S, Roblin G, Williams A, et al. Validity of sleep nasendoscopy in the investigation of sleep related breathing disorders. Laryngoscope 2005;115:538–40.
47. Rabelo FA, Braga A, Küpper DS, et al. Propofol-induced sleep: polysomnographic evaluation of patients with obstructive sleep apnea and controls. Otolaryngol Head Neck Surg 2010;142:218–24.
48. Eichler C, Sommer JU, Stuck BA, et al. Does drug-induced sleep endoscopy change the treatment concept of patients with snoring and obstructive sleep apnea? Sleep Breath 2012. [Epub ahead of print].
49. Campanini A, Canzi P, De Vito A, et al. Awake versus sleep endoscopy: personal experience in 250 OSAHS patients. Acta Otorhinolaryngol Ital 2010;30:73–7.
50. Kezirian EJ. Nonresponders to pharyngeal surgery for obstructive sleep apnea: insights from drug-induced sleep endoscopy. Laryngoscope 2011;121:1320–6.
51. Johal A, Hector MP, Battagel JM, et al. Impact of sleep nasendoscopy on the outcome of mandibular advancement splint therapy in subjects with sleep-related breathing disorders. J Laryngol Otol 2007;121:668–75.
52. Hohenhorst W, Ravesloot MJL, Kezirian EJ, et al. Drug-induced sleep endoscopy in adults with sleep-disordered breathing: technique and the VOTE classification system. Oper Tech Otolaryngol Head Neck Surg 2012;23:11–8.
53. Jacobowitz O. Perioperative management of patients with sleep-related breathing disorder. In: Wardrop P, Yaremchuk K, editors. Sleep medicine. San Diego (CA): Plural Publishing; 2010. p. 323–38.
54. Kezirian EJ, Weaver EM, Yueh B, et al. Risk factors for serious complication after uvulopalatopharyngoplasty. Arch Otolaryngol Head Neck Surg 2006;132:1091–8.
55. Osnes T, Rollheim J, Hartmann E. Effect of UPPP with respect to site of pharyngeal obstruction in sleep apnoea: follow-up at 18 months by overnight recording of airway pressure and flow. Clin Otolaryngol Allied Sci 2002;27:38–43.
56. Saigusa H, Yamashita K, Tanuma K, et al. Morphological studies for retrusive movement of the human adult tongue. Clin Anat 2004;17:93–8.
57. Jacobowitz O. Palatal and tongue base surgery for surgical treatment of obstructive sleep apnea: a prospective study. Otolaryngol Head Neck Surg 2006;135:258–64.
58. Pang KP, Woodson BT. Expansion sphincter pharyngoplasty: a new technique for the treatment of obstructive sleep apnea. Otolaryngol Head Neck Surg 2007;137:110–4.
59. Cahali MB, Formigoni GG, Gebrim EM, et al. Lateral pharyngoplasty versus uvulopalatopharyngoplasty: a clinical, polysomnographic and computed tomography measurement comparison. Sleep 2004;27:942–50.
60. Shine NP, Lewis RH. The "Propeller" incision for transpalatal advancement pharyngoplasty: a new approach to reduce post-operative oronasal fistulae. Auris Nasus Larynx 2008;35:397–400.
61. Friedman M, Ibrahim HZ, Vidyasagar R, et al. Z-palatoplasty(ZPP): a technique for patients without tonsils. Otolaryngol Head Neck Surg 2004;131:89–100.

62. Li HY, Lee LA. Relocation pharyngoplasty for obstructive sleep apnea. Laryngoscope 2009;119:2472–7.
63. Woodson BT. Innovative technique for lingual tonsillectomy and midline posterior glossectomy for obstructive sleep apnea. Oper Tech Otolaryngol Head Neck Surg 2007;18:20–8.
64. Riley RW, Powell NB, Guilleminault C. Inferior sagittal osteotomy of the mandible with hyoid myotomy-suspension: a new procedure for obstructive sleep apnea. Otolaryngol Head Neck Surg 1986;94:589–93.
65. Fibbi A, Ameli F, Brocchetti F, et al. Tongue base suspension and radiofrequency volume reduction: a comparison between 2 techniques for the treatment of sleep-disordered breathing. Am J Otolaryngol 2009;30:401–6.
66. Mickelson S. Hyoid advancement to the mandible (hyo-mandibular advancement). Oper Tech Otolaryngol Head Neck Surg 2012;23:56–9.
67. Holty JE, Guilleminault C. Maxillomandibular advancement for the treatment of obstructive sleep apnea: a systematic review and meta-analysis. Sleep Med Rev 2010;14:287–97.
68. Al-Bishri A, Rosenquist J, Sunzel B. On neurosensory disturbance after sagittal split osteotomy. J Oral Maxillofac Surg 2004;62:1472–6.
69. Kezirian EJ, Boudewyns A, Eisele DW, et al. Electrical stimulation of the hypoglossal nerve in the treatment of obstructive sleep apnea. Sleep Med Rev 2010; 14:299–305.
70. Eastwood PR, Barnes M, Walsh JH, et al. Treating obstructive sleep apnea with hypoglossal nerve stimulation. Sleep 2011;34:1479–86.

Medical Insurance for Dental Sleep Medicine

Marty R. Lipsey, DDS, MS

KEYWORDS

- Dental sleep medicine • Medical insurance • DME
- Oral appliance therapy

Over the last 5 to 7 years, I have observed many dental teams that have mastered the art and science of processing dental insurance for their patients but have major difficulties crossing the line and learning how to help their patients in this same process when it comes to medical insurance. This article is presented in an attempt to help resolve that problem and to provide a basic guide for the dental team in coding, billing, and processing of major medical insurance for dental sleep medicine. As with many other systems in our offices, there is not just one correct model. I present what I have come to call the "patient and physician friendly" model for dental sleep medicine—patient friendly because mastering this process allows the dental team to work with their patient's medical insurance carrier, allowing patients to minimize their up-front and total out-of-pocket expense, and physician friendly because mastering this process helps increase positive feedback from patients to their medical provider team, opening the door for further referrals.

By gaining a better understanding of medical insurance, what it will and will not cover, the dental team can be more accurate and more helpful in providing information to patients. Neither the patient nor the dental team welcomes any type of financial surprise. Understanding when medical insurance is and is not applicable helps everyone to be on the same page.

Many dental offices have adopted a medical insurance protocol of having patients pay in full up front and advising them to try to navigate the reimbursement maze on their own. This is certainly the patient and physician unfriendly model. I pose this question to you and your team, "If you help your patients with their dental insurance, why would you not want to educate yourselves so you can do the same with their medical insurance?" If your dental insurance protocol is not to process patients' dental insurance, then I see no conflict in doing the same on the medical side. Although there are some dental practices that follow this dental insurance model, I feel fairly confident in saying that it is the exception rather than the rule. If your dental patients have grown to expect that you provide this

Disclosure: I am the owner of Dental Sleep Med Systems, Inc, a California corporation specializing in consulting and practice management systems for dental sleep medicine.
3025 McHenry Avenue, Suite N, Modesto, CA 95350, USA
E-mail address: DrMarty@SnoringIsBoring.com

service, why not adopt the same patient-friendly model when it comes to their medical insurance? One of my goals is to help you to be able to do just that.

Working with physicians and the medical community is a must for expanding this area of practices. Without any regard to insurance, we need a medical diagnosis to properly treat this condition. Therefore, it should be evident from step 1 that we should strive to partner with our medical colleagues. In some cases that is easier said than done, but I think it should be a goal, nevertheless. One of the most often heard complaints from medical offices, and an easy way to put an end to these referrals before they really start, is to let these potential referrers hear from their patients that the dental office will not accept their medical insurance. Aside from cosmetic medical practices, there are very few medical offices that demand payment in full in advance. I would venture to say that dental offices are usually much more straightforward in making financial arrangements with patients before treatment than the average medical practice. The protocol of making sound written financial arrangements for your dental sleep medicine patients is certainly encouraged. The caveat here is that I would encourage you to make them in a patient and physician friendly manner.

Here is a true story that I hope will help to illustrate how one dental office did not see the big picture in terms of a physician and patient friendly model when it came to medical insurance for dental sleep medicine. Dr X, DDS, informed me that he had a great relationship with a medical office that was regularly referring patients with sleep apnea to him for oral appliance therapy (OAT). He was very happy that the physician was a strong believer in oral appliances (OAs) and routinely referred patients to him for this treatment option. Dr X was confident that I was wrong in promoting how his office should take a more proactive position in helping patients with their medical insurance. Dr X's policy was to ask for a payment of $2500 in advance and offer paperwork to patients to send in to their medical insurance carrier for possible reimbursement. Dr X proudly informed me that he had almost 100% case acceptance from all the patients who were referred from the physician's office. The situation was discussed in detail, and, when Dr X had a staff member call the referring medical office, they found the true situation. The medical office was aware of the approximate out-of-pocket cost to patients at Dr X's office for OAT. The referring medical office routinely informed their patients that they would have to pay this sum in advance if they wanted to consider this treatment option. The phone call to the medical office quickly revealed that less than one-third of the patients wanted the referral when they found out the costs involved and the insurance policy at Dr X's office. The 100% case acceptance was probably closer to a maximum of 30% when Dr X realized that the medical team was in effect financially screening patients before the referral was ever made. How much more effective could this referral source have been if the message to the patients was that Dr X's office will work with your medical insurance to make the treatment as affordable as possible? Is not that better marketing and more of what we would want for our patients if the shoe were on the other foot?

THE CENTERS FOR MEDICARE AND MEDICAID SERVICES 1500 FORM

Let us take a look at the form that was created by the Centers for Medicare and Medicaid Services (CMS, a branch of the US Department of Health and Human Services) and is the universal form for processing medical insurance for both Medicare and private payers for dental sleep medicine (**Fig. 1**).

Known as the CMS 1500 Form, this insurance form is used to process medical claims for both private payers and Medicare. Fields 1 to 13 are fairly intuitive and are completed using basic patient and doctor information. **Table 1** lists some comments on the remainder of the fields.

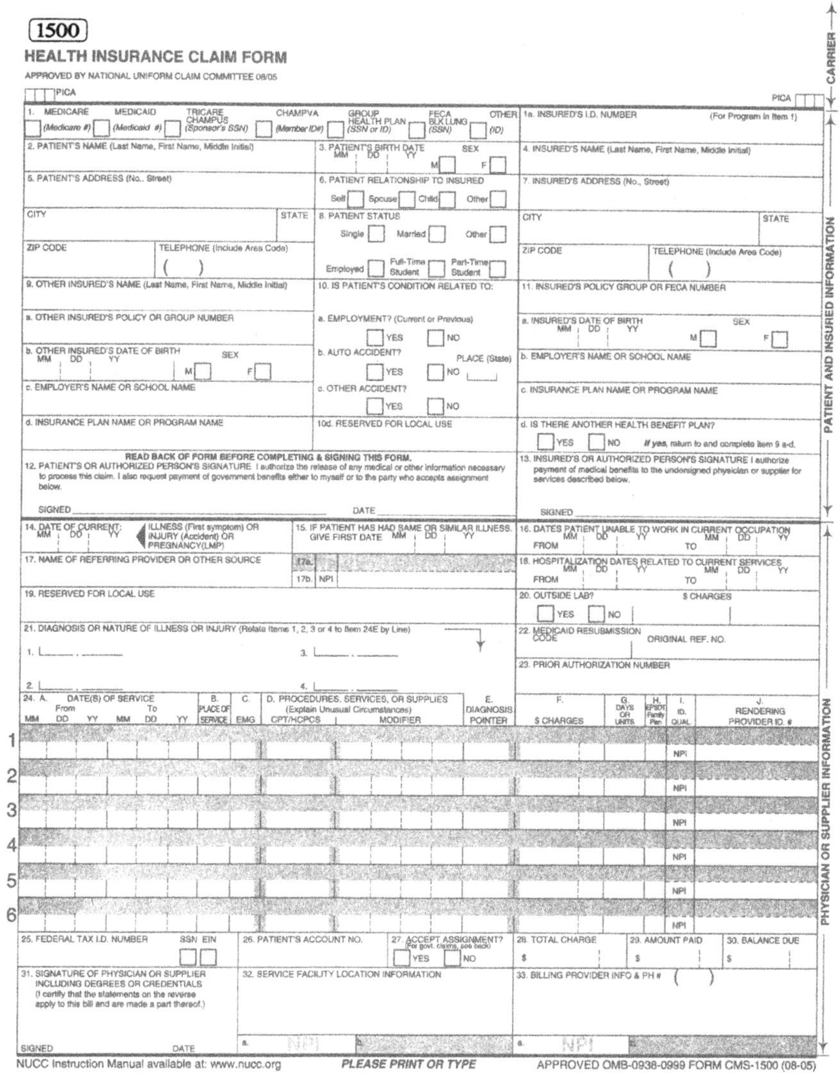
1500

HEALTH INSURANCE CLAIM FORM

APPROVED BY NATIONAL UNIFORM CLAIM COMMITTEE 08/05

PICA — PICA — CARRIER

1. MEDICARE (Medicare #) MEDICAID (Medicaid #) TRICARE CHAMPUS (Sponsor's SSN) CHAMPVA (Member ID#) GROUP HEALTH PLAN (SSN or ID) FECA BLK LUNG (SSN) OTHER (ID)

1a. INSURED'S I.D. NUMBER (For Program in Item 1)

2. PATIENT'S NAME (Last Name, First Name, Middle Initial)

3. PATIENT'S BIRTH DATE MM DD YY SEX M F

4. INSURED'S NAME (Last Name, First Name, Middle Initial)

5. PATIENT'S ADDRESS (No., Street)

6. PATIENT RELATIONSHIP TO INSURED Self Spouse Child Other

7. INSURED'S ADDRESS (No., Street)

CITY STATE

8. PATIENT STATUS Single Married Other

CITY STATE

ZIP CODE TELEPHONE (Include Area Code) ( )

Employed Full-Time Student Part-Time Student

ZIP CODE TELEPHONE (Include Area Code) ( )

9. OTHER INSURED'S NAME (Last Name, First Name, Middle Initial)

10. IS PATIENT'S CONDITION RELATED TO:

11. INSURED'S POLICY GROUP OR FECA NUMBER

a. OTHER INSURED'S POLICY OR GROUP NUMBER

a. EMPLOYMENT? (Current or Previous) YES NO

a. INSURED'S DATE OF BIRTH MM DD YY SEX M F

b. OTHER INSURED'S DATE OF BIRTH MM DD YY SEX M F

b. AUTO ACCIDENT? PLACE (State) YES NO

b. EMPLOYER'S NAME OR SCHOOL NAME

c. EMPLOYER'S NAME OR SCHOOL NAME

c. OTHER ACCIDENT? YES NO

c. INSURANCE PLAN NAME OR PROGRAM NAME

d. INSURANCE PLAN NAME OR PROGRAM NAME

10d. RESERVED FOR LOCAL USE

d. IS THERE ANOTHER HEALTH BENEFIT PLAN? YES NO *If yes, return to and complete item 9 a-d.*

READ BACK OF FORM BEFORE COMPLETING & SIGNING THIS FORM.

12. PATIENT'S OR AUTHORIZED PERSON'S SIGNATURE I authorize the release of any medical or other information necessary to process this claim. I also request payment of government benefits either to myself or to the party who accepts assignment below.

SIGNED DATE

13. INSURED'S OR AUTHORIZED PERSON'S SIGNATURE I authorize payment of medical benefits to the undersigned physician or supplier for services described below.

SIGNED

PATIENT AND INSURED INFORMATION

14. DATE OF CURRENT: MM DD YY ILLNESS (First symptom) OR INJURY (Accident) OR PREGNANCY(LMP)

15. IF PATIENT HAS HAD SAME OR SIMILAR ILLNESS. GIVE FIRST DATE MM DD YY

16. DATES PATIENT UNABLE TO WORK IN CURRENT OCCUPATION MM DD YY FROM TO

17. NAME OF REFERRING PROVIDER OR OTHER SOURCE 17a. 17b. NPI

18. HOSPITALIZATION DATES RELATED TO CURRENT SERVICES MM DD YY FROM TO

19. RESERVED FOR LOCAL USE

20. OUTSIDE LAB? YES NO $ CHARGES

21. DIAGNOSIS OR NATURE OF ILLNESS OR INJURY (Relate Items 1, 2, 3 or 4 to Item 24E by Line)

1. 2. 3. 4.

22. MEDICAID RESUBMISSION CODE ORIGINAL REF. NO.

23. PRIOR AUTHORIZATION NUMBER

24. A. DATE(S) OF SERVICE From To MM DD YY MM DD YY | B. PLACE OF SERVICE | C. EMG | D. PROCEDURES, SERVICES, OR SUPPLIES (Explain Unusual Circumstances) CPT/HCPCS MODIFIER | E. DIAGNOSIS POINTER | F. $ CHARGES | G. DAYS OR UNITS | H. EPSDT Family Plan | I. ID. QUAL. | J. RENDERING PROVIDER ID. #

1 NPI
2 NPI
3 NPI
4 NPI
5 NPI
6 NPI

PHYSICIAN OR SUPPLIER INFORMATION

25. FEDERAL TAX I.D. NUMBER SSN EIN

26. PATIENT'S ACCOUNT NO.

27. ACCEPT ASSIGNMENT? (For govt. claims, see back) YES NO

28. TOTAL CHARGE $

29. AMOUNT PAID $

30. BALANCE DUE $

31. SIGNATURE OF PHYSICIAN OR SUPPLIER INCLUDING DEGREES OR CREDENTIALS (I certify that the statements on the reverse apply to this bill and are made a part thereof.)

SIGNED DATE

32. SERVICE FACILITY LOCATION INFORMATION a. NPI b.

33. BILLING PROVIDER INFO & PH # ( ) a. NPI b.

NUCC Instruction Manual available at: www.nucc.org *PLEASE PRINT OR TYPE* APPROVED OMB-0938-0999 FORM CMS-1500 (08-05)

Fig. 1. CMS 1500 health insurance claim form.

CURRENT PROCEDURAL TERMINOLOGY/HEALTHCARE COMMON PROCEDURE CODING SYSTEM CODES

Current Procedural Terminology, or *CPT*, codes are a set of codes maintained by the American Medical Association to describe medical, surgical, and diagnostic services. The Healthcare Common Procedure Coding System is a set of health care procedure codes based on *CPT*. Visit codes, imaging codes, coding for pharyngometry and rhinometry, and the codes used for OAs all fall within these categories.

THE *INTERNATIONAL CLASSIFICATION OF DISEASES, NINTH REVISION*, CODES

The *International Classification of Diseases, Ninth Revision*, (*ICD-9*) is the official system of codes used in the United States to classify and assign codes to health

Table 1 CMS 1500 fields	
Field Number	**Comments**
1–13	Enter the applicable patient information
14	NA
15	NA
16	NA
17, 17a, 17b	NA
18	NA
19	NA
20	NA
21	Enter the patient's diagnosis/condition; must use an *ICD-9* diagnosis code number; you may enter up to 4 codes in priority order
22	NA
23	Enter preauthorization number if available
24A	Enter the date of service; the "From" and "To" date will usually be the same
24B	For code E0486, place of service is 12 (home) and all other office services rendered in the office are 11
24C	NA
24D	Enter the appropriate CPT/HCPCS code; Medicare requires the modifier NU for E0486; this modifier can be used universally
24E	Enter the diagnosis code reference number as shown in field 21 to relate the date of service and the procedures performed with the primary diagnosis; when multiple diagnoses are related to one service, the reference number for the primary diagnosis should be listed first; other applicable diagnosis reference numbers should follow
24F	Enter the charge for each listed service
24G	Enter the number of units; this field cannot be left blank and will usually be entered as "1"
24H	NA
24I	NA
24J	Enter rendering provider's NPI number
25	Enter tax ID number and check appropriate box
26	Not a required field, enter if you wish to specify a patient's account number
27	Required by Medicare and can be filled in for private payers as well
28	Enter total of column F
29	Enter total amount that patient has paid on covered services
30	Enter the difference between field 28 and field 29, not required by Medicare
31	Enter signature and date (can be entered digitally)
32	Enter name and address of facility where services were rendered
32a	Enter NPI number of service facility listed in 32
32b	NA
33	Enter physician/supplier billing name, address, zip code, and phone number
33a	Enter NPI number of entity listed in 33

Abbreviations: CPT/HCPCS, *Current Procedural Terminology*/Healthcare Common Procedure Coding System; *ICD-9*, *International Classification of Diseases, Ninth Revision*; ID, identification; NPI, National Provider Identifier.

conditions. In simpler terms, these are the codes that signify the disease, problem, or malady that we are treating. The most common *ICD-9* code in dental sleep medicine is for obstructive sleep apnea, which is 327.23. A dentist or dental team can only use this code when a physician has previously made that diagnosis.

DEDUCTIBLES

When we wear our dental hats, we are accustomed to dental insurance deductibles in the $50 to $150 range. Donning our medical hats, we have to be open to considering deductibles for medical insurance that can range to $5000 and sometimes even higher.

Deductibles are one of the top priority items on our checklist when we call to check benefits with a patient's medical insurance carrier. We recommend getting the following minimal list of information on deductibles:

1. What is the deductible amount?
2. Is the deductible based on a calendar year or otherwise?
3. How much of the current deductible has been satisfied?
4. Is there a specific durable medical equipment (DME) deductible?

Some medical insurance carriers have a deductible specific to DME. Although the OA is by definition DME, it is essential to know when a deductible may apply specifically to this area.

Patients with high deductibles, which have not been satisfied, may for all intents and purposes, actually become cash-paying/out-of-pocket–paying patients for OAT. The patient-friendly model involves advising the patient of such possibilities and still assisting by submitting everything to their medical carrier. Patients should be advised that you are submitting the treatment on their behalf, which will help them satisfy their deductible, should they need to use their medical benefits for other care during that same deductible-covered year.

IN-NETWORK VERSUS OUT-OF-NETWORK

Most dentists will be out of network when it comes to medical carriers. When calling to verify medical insurance benefits, the medical insurance company is not obligated to give you the full detail, in terms of the patient's insurance benefits, that it would provide to a physician who is a network provider for that same insurance company. Until your practice has received a sufficient number of payments from local medical carriers and has built a database of benefit information that you can use as a reference, you will need to use your best judgment to make sound financial arrangements for dental sleep medicine procedures with the patient. This does not imply that you should ask for full payment in advance. Our recommendation is that you gather as much information as possible from the medical insurance carrier and work with the patient to base the financial arrangement on that information.

It is not always a blessing to be in network. Some medical carriers have extremely low benefits for OAs, and out-of-network offices may actually get a higher level of benefit for the OA than a network provider. In some states, it is not possible for a dentist to be in network with major medical carriers.

On occasion, when you call a patient's medical insurance carrier to obtain insurance information for OAT, you may be told that there are no out-of-network benefits payable. In these instances, the best first course of action may be to ask who the in-network provider is for your geographic area. Be specific in asking for a provider that provides services for the procedure that corresponds to code E0486 (a custom fabricated oral device/appliance used to reduce upper airway collapsibility). More times than not, a telephone call to the office you have been provided information for will establish that this office does not actually provide OAT for sleep apnea. If that is the case, you would want to make a second call to the insurance company and request an out-of-network exception or gap exclusion from the medical carrier. This exception/exclusion is a method of asking the medical carrier to treat you as an in-network provider (without your having to contract as such) for the particular case. Because the patient does not have a network provider for OAT in your geographic area, it is usual (although sometimes an involved request) that the medical insurance carrier approve your providing care to the patient at a negotiated rate. The insurance carriers will outline their procedure for requesting this exclusion, which is usually done as a written follow-up. On the other hand, if your call to the in-network provider verifies that they do provide these dental sleep medicine services, the medical insurance carrier is fully within their right to advise you that they will not pay any benefits for the services unless rendered through their provider.

MEDICARE

Dental teams usually have many questions about Medicare. Dental sleep medicine is usually a dental team's first entry into the Medicare world. Medicare usually has no part in our dental practices, with the possible exception of some oral surgery practices or practices that may have a special oral surgery niche. Both Medicaid and Medicare are administered by the CMS. Medicaid is not part of this discussion because they do not have benefits for or administer OAT in any way, shape, or form.

Medicare views the dentist involved in dental sleep medicine as both a provider and a DME supplier. The procedures for becoming a Medicare part B provider are not the same as becoming a Medicare DME supplier. Also, there are different rules when it comes to treating Medicare beneficiaries in your office for part B evaluation and management procedures as compared with delivering the actual appliance when you are deemed a DME supplier.

The Dentist as a Provider

As a provider, to see Medicare beneficiaries and bill for evaluation and management procedures (office visits, testing procedures such as pharyngometry and rhinometry, and imaging), the dentist must register as a Medicare part B provider or opt out of Medicare part B. To register as a Medicare part B provider, you should complete a CMS-855I form and submit this form to the appropriate Medicare fee-for-service contractor serving your state. To opt out of Medicare part B, Medicare provides the following guidelines of what you must do: (1) notify your patients that you are opting out of Medicare; (2) file an affidavit with each carrier that has jurisdiction over the claims that you would otherwise file with Medicare; (3) enter into a private contract for, and before, rendering any covered services to a Medicare part B beneficiary; (4) install procedures to ensure that your office never files a Medicare claim and never provides information to patients that enables them to file a Medicare claim; and (5) mark your calendar to send in a new opt out affidavit every 2 years to maintain your status.

On the provider side, there may be examination and imaging services that are payable to a part B Medicare provider dentist for services rendered before the start of OAT. From my point of view, it is a matter of fact that dentists have to examine the patient, which may include testing and imaging, before determining if the patient is a candidate for OAT. Therefore, it follows that these services are not an actual part of the OAT regimen and should be billed and paid separately by Medicare part B. In the later section, you will be introduced to the concept of DME Medicare administrative contractors (DME MACs) and its definition of a bundled fee.

The Dentist as a Supplier

The OA, itself, is considered DME. As a DME, the appliance is billed to the appropriate DME MAC. Each DME MAC pays an all-inclusive bundled fee for the appliance and initial 90-day course of OAT. Palmetto GBA has published the following regarding this all-inclusive bundled fee, " …any radiological or other services performed to guide the adjustments of the oral device should not be submitted separately to the A/B MAC, as the Medicare payment associated with HCPCS code E0486 already includes any required adjustments to ensure a properly fitted device." There are 4 DME MACs that cover the United States, shown in **Fig. 2**, **Table 2**. To provide a custom fit OA to a Medicare beneficiary, you should follow 1 of the 2 procedures:

1. Register as a Medicare DME supplier with CMS by completing a CMS-855S form and submit this form to the National Supplier Clearinghouse that handles this application for all 4 DME MACs. A fee of $523 must be submitted online, and a copy of that payment should be submitted with your CMS-855S form. Medicare pays a bundled fee, determined by the jurisdiction your practice is located in, for the first 90 days of OAT. If you agree to accept this Medicare allowed fee as payment in full, the patient usually has no out of pocket expense. This fee is paid by electronic deposit to your pre-designated bank account.
2. Do not register with CMS as a DME Supplier. If you are not registered as a DME supplier with the Medicare system, you cannot bill Medicare for the oral appliance. Patients that are Medicare beneficiaries are allowed a once in a lifetime benefit to be reimbursed for expenses they incur through a non Medicare DME supplier. Therefore, in this situation, you can charge the patient your usual and customary fee for the oral appliance, including the first 90 days of care. The patient can

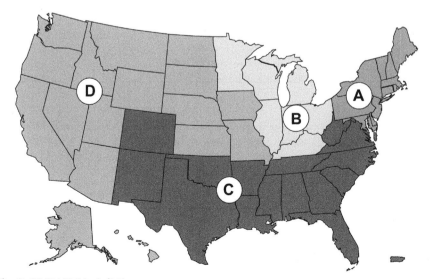

Fig. 2. DME MAC jurisdictions.

Table 2 DME MACs	
Jurisdiction A (National Heritage Insurance)	**Jurisdiction C (CIGNA Government Services)**
Connecticut	Alabama
Delaware	Arkansas
District of Columbia	Colorado
Maine	Florida
Maryland	Georgia
Massachusetts	Louisiana
New Hampshire	New Mexico
New Jersey	Mississippi
New York	North Carolina
Pennsylvania	Oklahoma
Rhode Island	South Carolina
Vermont	Tennessee
	Texas
	Virginia
	West Virginia
	Puerto Rico
	Virgin Islands
Jurisdiction B (National Government Services)	**Jurisdiction D (Noridian)**
Illinois	Alaska
Indiana	American Samoa
Kentucky	Arizona
Michigan	California
Minnesota	Guam
Ohio	Hawaii
Wisconsin	Idaho
	Iowa
	Kansas
	Missouri
	Montana
	Nebraska
	Nevada
	North Dakota
	Northern Mariana Islands
	Oregon
	South Dakota
	Utah
	Washington
	Wyoming

then apply to Medicare for reimbursement at the Medicare allowed rate. After the initial 90 days, you cannot charge a Medicare beneficiary for any follow up care unless you are a Medicare Part B provider or have opted out of Part B Medicare (see previous section).

On submitting either of these applications (855I or 855S), Medicare will, by default, assume you want to register as a nonparticipating provider. If you wish to be a participating provider, you must submit a CMS460 form along with your application.

As a nonparticipating provider, you retain the right to accept assignment or to not accept assignment on a case-by-case basis. This right is indicated on the CMS 1500 Form in field 27 for each claim you submit to Medicare. The method of Medicare payment to you as a nonparticipating provider follows the same formula as for part B and DME suppliers. If you accept assignment, Medicare will pay you 80% of the Medicare-approved fee. Either the patient's Medicare supplemental insurance or the patient pays the remaining 20%. If the patient does not have a supplemental insurance plan, you should collect the 20% balance from the patient. You are not allowed to charge the patient any amount beyond the Medicare-approved fee when you accept assignment.

If you are a nonparticipating provider and choose not to accept assignment from Medicare, payment in the amount of 80% of the Medicare-approved fee will go directly from Medicare to the patient. You are allowed to charge the patient a total fee, which is 15% more than the Medicare-approved fee.

If you are a participating provider, you must accept assignment on every case at the Medicare-approved fee. As a participating provider, Medicare directly pays you 80% of the approved fee. Either the patient's Medicare supplemental insurance or the patient pays the remaining 20%. If the patient does not have a supplemental insurance plan, you should collect the 20% balance from the patient. As a participating provider, you are not allowed to charge the patient beyond the Medicare-approved fee.

INSURANCE CONSIDERATIONS BEFORE OAT

Each office should develop a checklist and telephone routine to determine the patient's eligibility and medical insurance specifics before beginning OAT. A copy of the patient's medical insurance card should be kept in the patient record. Calling the customer service number given on the medical insurance card allows you to get vital information that will help in making a patient and physician friendly financial arrangement with the patient. The following is the minimum list of information you should get from the medical insurance carrier:

1. Annual deductible and amount satisfied
   a. Some medical insurance plans have very high deductibles. Patients will appreciate your submitting all claims to their medical insurance that should then be applied to their deductibles. However, when patients have a very high deductible, they will essentially become cash-paying patients, and you do not need any further specifics for your insurance checklist.
   b. Determine if deductibles are on a calendar year basis or otherwise.
   c. Determine if there is a specific DME deductible.
2. Requirement of precertification
   a. If precertification is required, you should find out the specifics for the payer and follow the procedure. Failure to follow this procedure, when it is a requirement, is almost a surefire denial when you submit for payment.
   b. If a precertification can be done by fax or the carrier is willing to give you a precertification number on the telephone, that is usually the quickest way to proceed.
3. Call reference number or agent identification (ID)
   a. The carrier records calls to customer service in the patient's insurance record. You should record this information in your permanent record. This is helpful, not only as a reference but also should you encounter any difficulty when subsequently filing the claim.
4. Restrictions on out-of-network benefits
   a. Most dental offices are not in-network with major medical insurance companies. As an out-of-network office, you will not be entitled to the same level of information when you call to get the patient's benefit information.

PUTTING IT ALL TOGETHER

I hope the information in this article assists your team to start or improve the ongoing process of helping patients say yes to OAT for obstructive sleep apnea. Although there is certainly a learning curve for the dental team in this endeavor, the patient and physician friendly dental sleep medicine practice is a model that will help to assure growth and success.

Appendix

ORGANIZATIONS OF INTEREST IN SLEEP MEDICINE FOR THE DENTIST

These are organizations that have a strong interest in sleep medicine and particularly as it relates to dental practice. All of them have annual meetings that are involved with sleep medicine and the treatment of sleep disorders.

American Academy of Sleep Medicine (AASM): A medical group that has a significant number of dentists as members.
Website: aasmnet.org
Address: 2510 North Frontage Road, Darien, Il 60561
Phone: 630-737-9700

American Academy of Dental Sleep Medicine (AADSM): The dental equivalent of the AASM and closely affiliated with them.
Website: www.aadsm.org
Address: 2510 North Frontage Road, Darien, Il 60561
Phone: 630-737-9761

The American Thoracic Society (ATS): An organization with a focus on pulmonary medicine that also has a large interest in sleep medicine.
Website: atsinfo@thoracic.org
Address: 25 Broadway – 18th Floor, New York, NY 10004
Phone: 212-315-8600

American College of Chest Physicians (AACP): A group made up of Pulmonologists that has an interest in sleep medicine as well.
Website: www.chestnet.org
Address: 3300 Dundee Road, Northbrook, IL 60062-2348
Phone: 847-498-1400

American Academy of Orofacial Pain (AAOP): An organization of primarily dentists with advanced training in orofacial pain and TMD with a strong interest and growing involvement in sleep medicine mainly because of the bidirectional relationship between chronic pain, headache and sleep disorders.
Website: www.aaop.org
Address: 174 South New York Avenue, PO Box 478, Oceanville, NJ 08231
Phone: 609-504-1311

Textbooks of Interest

These are textbooks that would be helpful and ones that any dentist who chooses to become more involved in sleep medicine may wish to read. There are many others that

Dent Clin N Am 56 (2012) 485–486
doi:10.1016/j.cden.2012.03.001
0011-8532/12/$ – see front matter © 2012 Published by Elsevier Inc.

dental.theclinics.com

are more comprehensive and would be valuable as ones experience and training expands.

The Promise of Sleep
   Author: William Dement, MD, PhD
   Available from bookstores and online publishers
   Publisher: Delacorte Press

Dental Management of Sleep Disorders
   Authors: R. Attanasio and DR Bailey
   Available from Wiley-Blackwell – www.wiley.com

Sleep Medicine for Dentists A Practical Overview
   Authors: GJ Lavigne, PA Cistulli, MT Smith
   Available from Quintessence Publishing – www.quintpub.com

Oral-Appliance Therapy in Obstructive Sleep Apnea-Hypopnea Syndrome
   A clinical study on therapeutic outcomes
   Author: Aarnoud Hoekema
   Available from the AADSM (see organizations)

Sleep Medicine Essentials
   Author: Teofilo Lee-Chiong
   Available from Wiley-Blackwell – 800-762-2974

Other Organizations – Websites of Interest

These are other areas that could be explored, most of whom are easily accessible on the internet.

National Sleep Foundation
   Website: www.sleepfoundation.org
   Located in Washington, DC

American Sleep Apnea Association
   Website: www.sleepapnea.org
   Located in Washington, DC

Talk About Sleep
   Website: www.talkaboutsleep.com

Index

Note: Page numbers of article titles are in **boldface** type.

Dent Clin N Am 56 (2012) 487–493
doi:10.1016/S0011-8532(12)00024-9
0011-8532/12/$ – see front matter © 2012 Elsevier Inc. All rights reserved.

dental.theclinics.com

Moving?

Make sure your subscription moves with you!

To notify us of your new address, find your **Clinics Account Number** (located on your mailing label above your name), and contact customer service at:

Email: journalscustomerservice-usa@elsevier.com

800-654-2452 (subscribers in the U.S. & Canada)
314-447-8871 (subscribers outside of the U.S. & Canada)

Fax number: 314-447-8029

Elsevier Health Sciences Division
Subscription Customer Service
3251 Riverport Lane
Maryland Heights, MO 63043

*To ensure uninterrupted delivery of your subscription, please notify us at least 4 weeks in advance of move.

Announcing
Dental **Advance**

The new, online home just for dentistry professionals

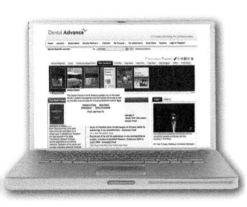

DentalAdvance.org is the gateway offering high-quality **research, news, jobs** and more for the **global community** of dental professionals.

What you'll find at DentalAdvance.org

- Journal profiles with quick links to **Tables of Contents, author submission** information, and subscription details
- Important information and valuable resources on how to submit a journal article
- Dentistry **Articles in Press** from participating journals
- Quick links to the leading dentistry societies worldwide
- **Dentistry News** from Elsevier Global Medical News (formerly IMNG)
- **Dentistry Jobs** powered by ElsevierHealthCareers.com

Bookmark us!
Visit DentalAdvance.org today.

Journals You'll Find At DentalAdvance.org
Dental Materials | Journal of Endodontics | Journal of Evidence-Based Dental Practice | Dental Abstracts | Dental Clinics of North America | Journal of Dental Sciences | Journal of Dentistry | The Saudi Dental Journal | Archives of Oral Biology | Oral Surgery, Oral Medicine, Oral Pathology, Oral Radiology, and Endodontics | American Journal of Orthodontics and Dentofacial Orthopedics | Mondo Ortodontico | Progress in Orthodontics | Seminars in Orthodontics | The Journal of Prosthetic Dentistry

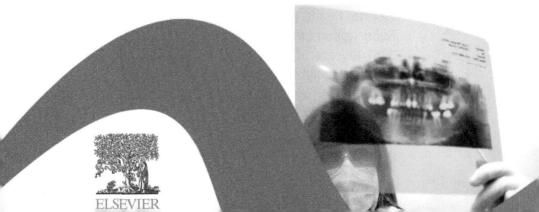

ELSEVIER

Printed and bound by CPI Group (UK) Ltd, Croydon, CR0 4YY

03/10/2024

01040455-0016